The Compassionate Core

Integrating Polyvagal Theory and Internal
Family Systems to Heal Complex Trauma
Step by Step

Landry Jerome Humphrey

This book is intended for educational and informational purposes only and should not be considered a substitute for professional medical advice, diagnosis, or treatment. Always seek the advice of your physician, licensed mental health professional, or other qualified health provider with any questions you may have regarding a medical or psychological condition. Never disregard professional medical advice or delay in seeking it because of something you have read in this book.

The techniques and suggestions presented in this book are not intended to replace proper medical or psychological treatment.. If you are currently in therapy, consult with your therapist before implementing any techniques from this book. If you are experiencing severe psychological distress, suicidal thoughts, or are in crisis, please contact your local emergency services immediately or call the National Suicide Prevention Lifeline.

All case examples and client stories in this book are composites drawn from multiple sources and extensively modified to protect privacy. Any resemblance to actual persons, living or dead, or actual events is purely coincidental. Names, characteristics, places, and incidents are products of the author's experience and imagination and are used fictitiously. The mention of specific organizations, therapists, researchers, or treatment modalities does not imply endorsement by those parties of this book's content.

The author and publisher disclaim any liability, loss, or risk, personal or otherwise, that is incurred as a consequence, directly or indirectly, of the use and application of any of the contents of this book. Readers are solely responsible for their own actions and decisions based on the information provided. This book is sold with the understanding that neither the author nor publisher is engaged in rendering psychological, medical, or other professional services.

Table of Contents

Introduction: The "Stuck" Survivor

You've already read the books.

Maybe it was *The Body Keeps the Score*. Or something about mindfulness. Or boundaries. Or attachment styles. You've highlighted passages, taken notes, nodded along, and thought, "Yes, that's me. That's exactly what I need."

And then... nothing changed.

Not really. Not in the ways that matter.

You still wake up with that knot in your stomach. You still freeze when someone raises their voice. You still find yourself scrolling through your phone at 2 AM, trying to numb the anxiety that won't let you sleep. You still feel like you're watching your life from behind glass—present but not really *there*.

Here's what nobody tells you: **Knowledge alone doesn't heal trauma.**

Understanding why you're anxious doesn't stop the panic attacks. Knowing your childhood was difficult doesn't make you feel less broken. Recognizing your patterns doesn't magically give you the power to change them.

And honestly? That's not your fault.

The problem isn't that you haven't tried hard enough or read enough or wanted it badly enough. The problem is simpler and more fixable than you think: **You've been trying to heal your mind while your body is still stuck in survival mode.**

Think about it. You sit down to journal about your feelings, and suddenly you're numb. You can't access anything. Or you try to meditate, and your thoughts race faster than ever. You want to

1

process that painful memory from childhood, but the moment you get close to it, you either shut down completely or spiral into a full-blown panic attack.

This isn't resistance. This isn't you "not wanting to heal." This is your nervous system doing its job—keeping you alive the only way it knows how.

The Missing Piece

Most trauma healing approaches focus on either the body *or* the mind. You'll find books about breathwork and yoga (body-focused) or books about cognitive reframing and parts work (mind-focused). Both are helpful. Both are necessary.

But here's the truth: **They only work when they work together.**

Your body and mind aren't separate systems. They're constantly communicating, constantly influencing each other. When your nervous system is in a state of threat—when your body is screaming "Danger!"—your mind can't do the healing work you're asking it to do. It's like trying to have a therapy session while someone is chasing you with a knife. Your brain has more urgent priorities.

This is where the **Compassionate Core** concept comes in.

Your Compassionate Core is the calm, clear, connected part of you that can actually heal. It's the part that can be curious instead of judgmental. Compassionate instead of critical. Present instead of panicked.

But (and this is the part most people miss) **you can only access your Compassionate Core when your body feels safe.**

Not when your nervous system *should* feel safe. Not when logically you know you're safe. When your nervous system actually, genuinely registers safety in your body.

This book brings together two powerful frameworks that, when combined, create a complete map for trauma healing:

Polyvagal Theory teaches you how to recognize and regulate your body's nervous system states. It explains why sometimes you're anxious, sometimes you're numb, and sometimes (rarely) you actually feel okay. More than that, it gives you practical tools to shift out of survival states and into that window of safety where healing becomes possible.

Internal Family Systems (IFS) teaches you how to work with the different "parts" of yourself—the inner critic, the perfectionist, the people-pleaser, the rage monster, the scared child. It shows you how to stop being at war with yourself and start leading from that Compassionate Core.

On their own, each approach is powerful. Polyvagal work helps you regulate your body, but doesn't always address the wounded parts that keep getting triggered. IFS helps you understand and heal those parts, but often fails when your nervous system is too dysregulated to access your compassionate Self.

Together, they're transformative.

Why This Book Is Different

This isn't another book that explains trauma theory and then leaves you wondering, "Okay, but what do I actually *do*?"

This is an integration manual. A step-by-step guide.

Every chapter builds on the one before it. You'll learn the theory you need (in plain language, without jargon), and then you'll get specific exercises, worksheets, and practices you can use immediately.

Here's the structure:

Part 1 gives you a new map for understanding trauma. You'll learn why you react the way you do, how your nervous system works, and why you have those conflicting voices in your head telling you different things. This section answers the "why" so you can stop blaming yourself and start seeing your symptoms as logical responses to what you've been through.

Part 2 gives you the five-step integration toolkit. These are the practical skills you'll use every single day. You'll learn how to:

1. Find your nervous system "anchor" (the felt sense of safety in your body)

2. Befriend your protective parts instead of fighting them

3. Work with the parts that try to rescue you through numbing or acting out

4. Safely witness and heal your wounded parts

5. Make decisions from your Compassionate Core

Part 3 shows you how to live with this new awareness. You'll get a troubleshooting guide for when you get triggered or stuck, and you'll learn how to move from just surviving to actually building a life you want to live.

Each chapter includes real examples. Not "a client once said" vague descriptions, but detailed scenarios that show you exactly how these concepts play out in real life. You'll see yourself in these stories. You'll recognize your patterns. And you'll start to understand that you're not broken—you're just using an outdated operating system that once kept you safe but now keeps you stuck.

What You Can Expect

This work isn't easy. Anyone who tells you healing happens quickly or painlessly is lying.

But it's simpler than you think.

You don't need years of therapy (though therapy can definitely help). You don't need to relive every traumatic memory in detail. You don't need to become a meditation expert or a psychology scholar.

You just need to learn how to recognize what state your body is in, how to gently shift toward safety, and how to compassionately work with the parts of yourself that are stuck in the past.

That's it. That's the whole process.

Does it take practice? Absolutely. Will you have setbacks? Of course. Healing isn't linear. Some days you'll feel like you're finally getting it, and the next day you'll be right back in old patterns.

But here's the difference: **You'll understand what's happening.** You'll have tools. You'll know how to find your way back.

And slowly, sometimes so slowly you don't even notice it happening, you'll spend less time in survival mode and more time in your Compassionate Core. You'll make choices you're proud of instead of choices you regret. You'll connect with people without constantly bracing for betrayal. You'll feel your feelings without being overwhelmed by them.

You'll heal. Not perfectly. Not completely. But enough to live the life you deserve.

A Word of Caution

This book is about integration—bringing your body and mind together so they can work as a team. That means you can't skip ahead to the "good parts." You can't just read Chapter 8 about healing your wounded parts and expect it to work if you haven't learned how to regulate your nervous system first.

So do yourself a favor: Read this in order. Do the exercises. Take your time with the worksheets. This isn't a race.

Your nervous system has been protecting you for years, maybe decades. It's not going to change overnight just because you read a chapter. But with consistent practice, with self-compassion, with patience—it will change.

And when it does, everything else changes too.

You just need to learn how to recognize what state your body is in, how to gently shift towards safety, and how to compassionately work with the parts of yourself that are stuck in the past.

That's it. That's the whole process.

Do it in real practice. Absolutely. Will you have setbacks? Of course. Healing isn't linear. Some days you'll feel like you're finally getting it, and the next day you'll be right back in old patterns.

But here's the difference: You'll understand what's happening. You'll have tools. You'll know how to find your way back.

And slowly, sometimes so slowly you don't even notice it happening, you'll spend less time in survival mode and more time in your Compassionate Core. You'll make choices you're proud of, instead of reactions you regret. You'll connect with people without constantly bracing for betrayal. You'll feel your feelings without being overwhelmed by them.

You'll heal. Not perfectly, but completely enough to live the life you want.

A Word of Caution

This book moves a little fast. It will teach you tools and mind... as you... conversations... practice... understand at all... You can't... later on. Chapter 8 must... Simply put, the nervous system will especially if you haven't learned how to regulate your nervous system first.

So do yourself a favor. Read this in order. Let the chapters sink. Take your time with the worksheets. This is a process.

Your nervous system has built protections that for years, maybe decades. It's not going to change overnight just because you read one chapter. But with consistent practice, with self-compassion, with patience—it will change.

And when it does, everything else change, too.

6

Chapter 1: A New Map for Trauma

You probably blame yourself.

Not for the trauma itself, maybe. You might intellectually understand that what happened to you wasn't your fault—whether it was abuse, neglect, chaos, or just the thousand small ways your needs went unmet.

But you blame yourself for how you are *now*.

For being too anxious. Too withdrawn. Too sensitive. Too reactive. For not being able to "just get over it" the way other people seem to. For still being affected by things that happened years ago.

You blame yourself for being stuck.

Here's what I need you to understand right from the start: **Your symptoms aren't character flaws. They're survival responses.**

Every single thing you do that frustrates you—the panic attacks, the emotional numbness, the people-pleasing, the angry outbursts, the inability to trust, the constant hypervigilance—all of it made perfect sense at some point in your life. All of it kept you safe when you needed protection.

The problem isn't that these responses exist. The problem is that they're still running even though the original threat is gone.

What Complex Trauma Actually Is

Let's start with a definition that actually makes sense.

Complex trauma (sometimes called C-PTSD or Complex Post-Traumatic Stress Disorder) isn't about one terrible event. It's about repeated, ongoing experiences that taught your nervous system: *The world is not safe. People are not trustworthy. I am not okay.*

These experiences usually happen early in life, often in childhood, and they usually involve the people who were supposed to take care of you (Herman, 1997).

Maybe your parent was unpredictable—loving one moment, rageful the next. You never knew which version you'd get. So you learned to scan for danger constantly, to read micro-expressions, to make yourself small and agreeable.

Or maybe your parent was absent—physically there but emotionally checked out. You learned that your needs didn't matter, that expressing feelings was pointless, that you had to handle everything alone.

Or maybe there was outright abuse—physical, sexual, emotional. You learned that your body wasn't yours, that pain was normal, that survival meant shutting down parts of yourself.

Or maybe it was more subtle. Maybe your family looked fine from the outside, but inside there was criticism, pressure, conditional love, emotional manipulation. You learned to perform, to achieve, to be perfect—because being yourself wasn't enough.

Here's the thing about complex trauma: **It fundamentally changes how your brain and body respond to the world** (van der Kolk, 2014).

Single-incident trauma (like a car accident or natural disaster) is different. It's terrible, but often people can process it and move on. Complex trauma rewires your system. It doesn't just give you memories to process—it changes your baseline. It affects how you experience safety, how you form relationships, how you regulate emotions, how you see yourself.

This isn't a life sentence. But it is a different starting point than someone who grew up with consistent safety and attunement. You're not broken. You're operating with different hardware, installed during a time when that hardware was absolutely necessary.

The Two Core Problems

When you're dealing with complex trauma, you're actually dealing with two interconnected problems:

Problem 1: You are hijacked by your nervous system.

Your body's alarm system is stuck in the "on" position. Even when you're objectively safe—sitting in your apartment, talking to a friend, lying in bed—your nervous system may be screaming that you're in danger.

This isn't psychological. This isn't "all in your head." This is physiological.

Your autonomic nervous system, which controls your stress response, has learned to default to threat states. It's like having a smoke detector that goes off when you toast bread. The detector is working perfectly—it's doing exactly what it was designed to do. It's just calibrated wrong.

So you go through life in states of high anxiety (fight-or-flight) or shutdown (freeze/collapse), rarely feeling calm and connected. Your body is preparing you to survive a threat that isn't actually there.

Problem 2: You are at war with your inner "parts."

At the same time, different aspects of your personality are in conflict.

Part of you wants to connect with people, but another part pushes them away. Part of you wants to feel your feelings, but another part numbs you out. Part of you wants to try new things, but another part keeps you playing it safe.

These aren't random contradictions. They're different survival strategies that developed at different times, for different threats. And

9

they're all trying to protect you—but they're not coordinating with each other.

It's like having a committee running your life, with each member shouting over the others, and nobody actually in charge.

Why Traditional Approaches Fall Short

You've probably tried therapy. Maybe it helped some. Maybe it didn't.

Traditional talk therapy was designed for single-event trauma. It assumes you can talk about what happened, make connections, gain insight, and then feel better. For complex trauma, that often doesn't work.

Why? Because when you try to talk about painful experiences, one of two things happens:

Option 1: You shut down. You feel numb, disconnected, like you're reading a script. You can describe what happened, but you don't feel anything. This is your body's dorsal vagal response—immobilization. Your nervous system has essentially pulled the plug to protect you from overwhelm.

Option 2: You get overwhelmed. Your heart races, you can't breathe, you feel like you're back in the trauma. You're not remembering what happened—you're reliving it. This is your sympathetic nervous system hijacking you.

In either state, you can't access the part of you that can actually heal—your calm, compassionate, curious Self.

So you keep talking about your trauma, keep trying to "process" it, but nothing shifts. Because you're trying to do mind-work (understanding, reframing, making meaning) while your body is in a survival state.

It's like trying to have a thoughtful conversation while running from a bear. Your body has other priorities.

The Way Forward

Here's the good news: There's a way through this that actually works.

You can rewire your nervous system. Your body can learn new responses. That smoke detector can be recalibrated. This isn't about positive thinking or willpower—it's about giving your nervous system repeated experiences of actual, embodied safety until it starts to believe that safety is possible (Porges, 2011).

You can integrate your parts. Those conflicting voices can learn to work together, with a wise, compassionate leader (your Self) coordinating them. This isn't about getting rid of parts or suppressing them—it's about helping them trust that you're no longer in the situation that created them (Schwartz, 2019).

But—and this is crucial—the body work has to come first.

You can't negotiate with your parts when your nervous system is in survival mode. Your protector parts won't step aside and let you access your wounded parts until they trust that you can handle it— and they only trust that when your body is regulated.

This is why this book teaches Polyvagal Theory *before* Internal Family Systems. Not because one is more important than the other, but because they work in a specific sequence.

First: Learn to recognize what state your nervous system is in.

Second: Learn to shift toward safety, even for brief moments.

Third: Once you can access a calm, connected state (even briefly), *then* you can start working with your parts.

This is the integration model. Body first, then mind. Regulation first, then transformation.

A Different Kind of Responsibility

So no, what happened to you wasn't your fault. You didn't choose your childhood. You didn't ask for the experiences that shaped you.

But here's the hard part: **What you do with it now is your responsibility.**

Not your fault, but your responsibility. There's a difference.

You can't change what happened. You can't get a do-over on your childhood. You can't make the people who hurt you suddenly show up differently.

But you can change how your nervous system responds. You can change how your parts interact. You can build the internal safety that you didn't get externally.

This isn't fair. You shouldn't have to do this work. If the world were just, you would have grown up safe and attuned, and none of this would be necessary.

But the world isn't fair. And waiting for it to be fair, or waiting for someone else to fix you, or waiting to feel ready—that's just staying stuck.

The path forward requires action. Not perfect action. Not massive action. Just consistent, compassionate action toward building a nervous system that can rest and a Self that can lead.

This book gives you the map. The walking is up to you.

Sarah's Story: Recognizing the Pattern

Sarah, a 34-year-old graphic designer, came to therapy exhausted. She'd been in therapy on and off for years, working on her "issues"—anxiety, relationship problems, perfectionism. She could articulate exactly why she had these issues. Her mother had been critical and dismissive. Her father had been absent. She'd learned to achieve her way to worth.

She understood all of this. She could explain it clearly to anyone who asked.

But understanding changed nothing. She still woke up with dread. Still spent hours obsessing over minor mistakes at work. Still pushed away anyone who tried to get close. Still felt fundamentally broken.

"I've read all the books," she said. "I know what my problem is. So why can't I just fix it?"

The breakthrough came when she learned about nervous system states. She started tracking when she felt anxious versus numb versus (rarely) calm. She noticed that she spent most of her time in sympathetic activation—her body constantly preparing for threat, even when she was safe.

More than that, she realized that when she tried to "work on herself"—journaling, meditating, trying to access compassion for her younger self—she was doing it from an activated state. Her body was in fight-or-flight mode while her mind tried to do healing work.

"It's like I was trying to perform surgery on myself while running a marathon," she said.

Once she learned to regulate her nervous system first—to find moments of genuine calm in her body—*then* she could access compassion for herself. Then she could work with the part that pushed people away and understand what it was protecting her from.

The work didn't get easier. But it finally started working.

What This Means for You

As you read this book, you're going to learn a new language for understanding yourself.

Instead of "I'm anxious," you'll learn to think "My sympathetic nervous system is activated."

Instead of "I'm a perfectionist," you'll learn to think "I have a manager part that tries to control everything to keep me safe."

13

Instead of "Why can't I just get over this?" you'll learn to think "What is my system trying to protect me from right now?"

This isn't just semantic. This is a fundamental shift in how you relate to your experience.

Your symptoms stop being evidence that you're broken and start being information about what your system needs. Your reactions stop being shameful and start being understandable. Your parts stop being the enemy and start being allies doing their best with limited information.

This shift in perspective is the foundation for everything else in this book.

You're not too damaged to heal. You're not too far gone. You're not uniquely broken.

You're a human being who survived difficult circumstances using the tools available to you at the time. Those tools worked then. They're not working now. So we're going to update your system with new tools—not by force, not by willpower, but by creating conditions where your nervous system can relax and your parts can rest.

That's the journey ahead.

What You Need to Move Forward

Here's what you need to get the most out of this book:

1. **Patience with yourself.** Your nervous system didn't get this way overnight. It won't change overnight. That's okay. Slow progress is still progress.

2. **Willingness to feel.** Not to drown in feelings, but to start noticing them. To stop numbing quite so aggressively. To stay present with discomfort without immediately trying to fix it.

3. **Curiosity instead of judgment.** When you notice yourself doing something you don't like—shutting down, lashing out, people-pleasing—get curious about it instead of beating yourself up. "Interesting. What's this about? What am I protecting myself from?"

4. **Practice.** You can't just read this and expect to change. You have to do the exercises, try the techniques, notice what happens in your body.

5. **Self-compassion.** You're going to mess up. You're going to forget what you've learned and fall back into old patterns. You're going to have bad days. That's part of the process. Shame doesn't help. Compassion does.

Can you bring these things to this work? Can you be patient and curious and willing to try?

If so, you're ready.

If not, that's okay too. But you might want to ask yourself what's in the way. Is it a part that's scared? Is it your nervous system trying to protect you from disappointment? Get curious about that. That's actually where the work begins.

Points to Remember

Complex trauma isn't a character flaw—it's a logical survival response to circumstances where you needed protection. Your symptoms aren't evidence you're broken; they're evidence that your system worked exactly as designed to keep you safe. The challenge now isn't that you're damaged beyond repair, but that your nervous system is still responding to threats that no longer exist.

You're dealing with two interconnected problems: a nervous system stuck in survival mode and internal parts that conflict with each other. Neither traditional talk therapy nor body-work alone can fully address this. You need both—but in the right order. Regulate the body first, then work with the parts.

This isn't about gaining more insight into why you're stuck. You probably already know why. This is about learning practical skills to shift your nervous system into safety and coordinate your parts from a place of calm, compassionate leadership. That's the difference between understanding your trauma and actually healing from it.

Chapter 2: The Body's Alarm System(Polyvagal Theory Made Simple)

Your body is talking to you. Right now.

It's sending signals about safety and threat, connection and danger, every single moment. The problem is, you probably can't hear it. Or when you do hear it, you don't trust it.

Maybe your body says you're in danger when you're objectively safe—sitting at your desk, driving to work, talking to a friend. Maybe it tells you to shut down and disappear when you actually need to speak up. Maybe it puts you on high alert for threats that aren't there and misses actual problems right in front of you.

Your body's alarm system isn't broken. It's just miscalibrated.

And once you understand how it works, you can start to recalibrate it.

This is where Polyvagal Theory comes in. Don't worry—I'm going to keep this simple. No neuroscience jargon. No complex diagrams. Just the essential information you need to understand what your body is doing and why.

The Nervous System You Didn't Know You Had

You probably learned in school that your nervous system has two parts: sympathetic (fight-or-flight) and parasympathetic (rest-and-digest). That's incomplete.

Dr. Stephen Porges discovered that the parasympathetic system actually has two branches that do completely different things (Porges, 2011). This changes everything about how we understand trauma and safety.

Here's what actually happens in your body:

Your autonomic nervous system runs constantly in the background, outside your conscious control. It regulates your heart rate, breathing, digestion, immune function—all the stuff that keeps you alive without you thinking about it.

But more than that, it's constantly scanning your environment for cues of safety and danger. This process, called *neuroception*, happens below your awareness (Porges, 2004). Your nervous system is making decisions about whether you're safe or threatened before your thinking brain even knows what's happening.

Based on what it detects, it shifts you into one of three core states. You move up and down this ladder throughout the day, often without noticing the transitions.

Let's look at each state.

State 1: Safe and Social (Ventral Vagal)

This is your Compassionate Core.

When your nervous system detects genuine safety—not just the absence of threat, but the active presence of cues that say "You're okay, you belong, you're connected"—it activates your ventral vagal system.

In this state, you feel:

- Calm and centered
- Socially engaged
- Curious and open
- Capable of thinking clearly
- Able to feel your emotions without being overwhelmed
- Connected to yourself and others

Your body in this state:

- Relaxed facial muscles (you can make eye contact, smile naturally)

- Smooth, easy breathing

- Warm hands and feet (good blood flow)

- Comfortable digestion

- A sense of presence in your body

This is the state where healing happens. This is where you can access compassion for yourself, curiosity about your parts, and the capacity to stay present with difficult feelings without spiraling.

But (and here's the key) **most trauma survivors spend very little time here.**

If you grew up in an environment where safety was rare or unpredictable, your nervous system never got much practice in this state. It doesn't know how to rest here. It feels unfamiliar, maybe even dangerous.

Some trauma survivors actually feel anxious when things are calm. Their nervous system has learned to expect the other shoe to drop, so stillness feels like the moment before the explosion.

State 2: Fight-or-Flight (Sympathetic)

When your nervous system detects threat—or thinks it detects threat—it mobilizes your body to deal with danger.

This is your sympathetic nervous system kicking in. It's designed for action: fight the threat or run from it.

In this state, you feel:

- Anxious, worried, panicked

- Angry, irritable, rageful

- Agitated, restless, unable to settle

- Obsessive, ruminating

- Hypervigilant (scanning for danger)

Your body in this state:

- Heart racing or pounding

- Rapid, shallow breathing

- Tense muscles, clenched jaw

- Cold hands and feet (blood to core for protection)

- Upset stomach or butterflies

- Trouble focusing or thinking clearly

This state isn't inherently bad. If there's an actual threat—a car swerving into your lane, a genuine emergency—this response is perfect. It gives you energy, speed, and focus to deal with danger.

The problem with complex trauma is that this state activates when there's no actual threat. Your nervous system perceives danger everywhere because it learned that danger *was* everywhere.

So you lie in bed worrying about everything. You snap at people who didn't do anything wrong. You catastrophize about minor problems. You can't relax because your body is convinced something bad is about to happen.

You're not anxious. Your nervous system is in sympathetic activation.

That's not just semantics. It shifts the whole approach. You can't think your way out of an activated nervous system. You have to work with your body to send it safety signals.

State 3: Shutdown (Dorsal Vagal)

If fight-or-flight doesn't work—if the threat is too big, too overwhelming, or inescapable—your nervous system has one more strategy: shut down.

This is your dorsal vagal system. It's an ancient survival mechanism, the same one that makes animals "play dead" when they can't escape a predator.

In this state, you feel:

- Numb, disconnected, foggy

- Depressed, hopeless, empty

- Exhausted beyond sleep

- Dissociated (watching yourself from outside)

- Unable to feel emotions or care about anything

Your body in this state:

- Low energy, heaviness

- Slow breathing and heart rate

- Collapsed posture

- Digestive issues (often constipation)

- Feeling cold or frozen

- Difficulty moving or speaking

This is often the most misunderstood state. People think it's depression or laziness or lack of motivation. But it's actually a protective response—your nervous system's last-ditch attempt to help you survive something unbearable.

If you couldn't fight or flee from trauma (especially in childhood when you were small and powerless), shutdown was the only option. Your system pulled the plug to protect you from overwhelming pain.

The problem is, this response keeps happening even when you're no longer powerless. Now, when life gets hard or emotions feel too big, your system still reaches for shutdown as its go-to strategy.

So you can't cry even though you want to. You feel nothing instead of the pain you need to feel. You can't seem to care about things that matter to you. You're present but not really there.

You're not lazy or numb. Your nervous system is in dorsal vagal shutdown.

Again, this isn't about blame. This is about understanding what's actually happening so you can work with it.

The Ladder: Moving Between States

Here's the key insight from Polyvagal Theory: **You move through these states in a specific order.**

Think of it as a ladder:

Top: Safe and Social (Ventral Vagal) When you feel safe, you're at the top—calm, connected, capable.

Middle: Fight-or-Flight (Sympathetic) When you perceive threat, you drop down into mobilization—anxious, agitated, ready to run.

Bottom: Shutdown (Dorsal Vagal) When threat becomes overwhelming, you drop to the bottom—immobilized, numb, gone.

You don't jump from the top to the bottom. You move through fight-or-flight on the way down.

And here's the critical part: **To get back to safety at the top, you have to move back up through fight-or-flight.**

This explains why, when you're shut down and numb, sometimes you need to feel anxious or angry as you move back toward regulation. That's not regression. That's your system climbing back up the ladder.

Marcus's Story: Living on the Ladder

Marcus, a 41-year-old accountant, described his life like this: "I'm either overwhelmed or I'm nothing. There's no middle ground."

At work, he was in constant fight-or-flight. Worrying about deadlines, imagining worst-case scenarios, checking and rechecking his work, sending tense emails late at night. His jaw hurt from clenching. He couldn't sleep. Every conversation with his boss felt like a threat.

Then, when he got home, he'd collapse. Not just tired—collapsed. He'd lie on the couch and scroll his phone for hours, feeling nothing. His wife would try to talk to him and he couldn't even respond. He was physically present but completely checked out.

"I don't enjoy anything anymore," he said. "I used to love working on my car, playing guitar. Now I just... exist."

When he learned about the nervous system states, everything clicked.

Work pushed him into sympathetic activation—his system perceived every deadline, every email, every interaction as a potential threat. He'd stay there for hours, his body pumping stress hormones, his mind racing with catastrophic thoughts.

Then, when the perceived threat passed (when he left the office), his system would crash into dorsal shutdown. He'd literally run out of gas. His body and brain would shut down to recover from the constant activation.

He wasn't choosing to be anxious at work or numb at home. His nervous system was doing what it was designed to do—cycling between mobilization and immobilization based on perceived threat.

The breakthrough came when he started catching these transitions. He'd notice: "I'm activated right now. My heart is racing. I'm catastrophizing. This is sympathetic."

Just naming it helped. It gave him a little distance, a little perspective. He could see that his anxious thoughts weren't reality—they were his nervous system's threat responses.

He started practicing finding his "ventral anchor"—we'll get to what that means in later chapters. For now, what matters is that he learned to recognize his states and gradually spend more time in safety instead of bouncing between alarm and collapse.

Why This Matters for Trauma

If you experienced complex trauma, your nervous system learned to default to threat states.

Maybe you ping-pong between sympathetic and dorsal—anxious and activated, then shut down and numb. Maybe you're stuck primarily in one state (constant anxiety or chronic shutdown). Maybe you have brief moments of ventral calm that get interrupted the moment anything stressful happens.

Here's what most people don't understand: **This isn't a psychological problem. This is a physiological one.**

Your nervous system isn't choosing to be difficult. It's responding to learned patterns. It genuinely believes you're in danger most of the time because, at one point, you were.

Those neural pathways got reinforced over and over—thousands of repetitions of "not safe, not safe, not safe." Now they're your default.

But here's the hopeful part: **Neural pathways can change** (Cozolino, 2017).

Your nervous system can learn new patterns. It can learn that calm is possible. That safety exists. That connection doesn't always lead to betrayal or hurt.

But it takes practice. Lots of practice. You're literally building new neural pathways, creating new defaults.

This isn't about positive thinking or willpower. It's about giving your nervous system repeated experiences of genuine, embodied safety until those new pathways become stronger than the old ones.

Mixed States and Complications

Sometimes you're in more than one state at once.

Maybe your body is in shutdown (heavy, frozen, numb) but your mind is in sympathetic activation (racing thoughts, worrying). This is exhausting—you're immobilized but not resting.

Or maybe you're in ventral socially (smiling, laughing, seeming fine) but there's sympathetic activation underneath (heart racing, stomach tight). This is what high-functioning anxiety looks like—capable on the outside, panicking on the inside.

These mixed states are common with complex trauma. Your system is trying to manage multiple things at once: stay safe, look normal, protect yourself, connect with others. It's doing its best. It's just complicated.

The Pull Toward Familiar States

Here's something nobody tells you: **Even unpleasant states can feel comfortable if they're familiar.**

If you grew up anxious, sympathetic activation might feel normal. Calm might feel strange, even threatening. Your system knows how to do anxiety. Anxiety is predictable. Safety is unknown territory.

Same with shutdown. If you spent your childhood dissociated, numbness might feel like home. Feeling your emotions might be terrifying.

This is why healing isn't just about getting to a better state. It's about learning to tolerate the unfamiliarity of that better state.

Your nervous system needs practice being calm. It needs to learn that calm doesn't mean you've let your guard down dangerously. It needs to experience, over and over, that you can be in your body, feeling your feelings, connected to others, and still be safe.

This is the work.

The Worksheet: Mapping Your States

Let's make this practical. You need to start noticing your patterns.

Over the next week, check in with yourself several times a day. Set a reminder on your phone if you need to. Ask yourself:

"What state is my nervous system in right now?"

Ventral (Safe and Social):

- Am I feeling calm, connected, and clear?
- Can I think without racing thoughts?
- Do I feel present in my body?
- Can I access curiosity or compassion?

Sympathetic (Fight-or-Flight):

- Is my heart racing?
- Am I feeling anxious, worried, or angry?
- Are my thoughts racing or looping?
- Am I scanning for threats?
- Do I feel restless or agitated?

Dorsal (Shutdown):

- Do I feel numb, foggy, or disconnected?
- Is it hard to think or make decisions?

26

- Do I feel heavy, frozen, or exhausted?

- Am I dissociated or checked out?

- Do I feel hopeless or empty?

Write down your observations. Don't judge them. Just notice.

Where do you spend most of your time?

If you're mostly in sympathetic, you're living in constant mobilization. If you're mostly in dorsal, you're living in chronic shutdown. If you bounce between them, you're exhausting your system with the back-and-forth.

The goal isn't to be in ventral all the time—that's not realistic. The goal is to spend more time there than you currently do, and to recognize when you've dropped into a threat state so you can help your system climb back up.

What triggers you into each state?

Notice patterns. Maybe certain people consistently push you into sympathetic. Maybe certain activities drop you into dorsal. Maybe certain environments feel safer and help you access ventral.

This information is gold. It tells you what your nervous system perceives as threatening and what it experiences as safe.

When you're in a threat state, how long do you stay there?

Hours? Days? Do you spiral and get stuck, or can you shift relatively quickly? This tells you about your nervous system's flexibility—its ability to move between states.

The more rigid your system (stuck in one state for long periods), the more practice you'll need building flexibility. The more you practice, the easier it gets to shift.

Understanding, Not Fixing

Right now, we're just building awareness. You're learning the language of your nervous system.

Don't try to fix anything yet. Don't judge yourself for being in "bad" states. Don't force yourself into ventral when your system isn't ready.

Just notice. Get curious. Build the muscle of paying attention to your body.

In the next chapters, you'll learn practical tools to work with each state. But first, you need to be able to recognize what state you're in.

You can't change what you can't see.

What You Now Understand

Your nervous system operates in three distinct states, not two. At the top is the ventral vagal state where you feel calm, connected, and capable—this is your Compassionate Core. In the middle is the sympathetic state where you're mobilized for threat through anxiety, anger, or agitation. At the bottom is the dorsal vagal state where you shut down into numbness, fog, and disconnection.

Your nervous system moves between these states based on neuroception—automatic, unconscious scanning for safety and danger. This happens below your awareness, which is why you can feel anxious when you're objectively safe or numb when you need to feel. Your body is responding to learned patterns, not current reality.

Complex trauma trains your nervous system to default to threat states. But these aren't permanent. Neural pathways can change with practice. The first step is simply learning to recognize which state you're in at any given moment, without judgment. You can't shift what you can't see, and awareness is where all change begins.

Chapter 3: The People Inside (Internal Family Systems Made Simple)

You are not one person.

That probably sounds strange. Maybe even concerning. But stay with me.

You're not "multiple personalities" in the clinical sense. You're a healthy person with different aspects of yourself that sometimes feel like they're pulling in opposite directions.

Part of you wants to speak up in meetings, but another part keeps you quiet. Part of you wants connection, but another part pushes people away. Part of you wants to feel your feelings, but another part numbs you out immediately.

These aren't contradictions in your personality. They're different *parts* of you, each with its own perspective, its own concerns, its own strategies for keeping you safe.

And right now, they're probably not working together very well.

The Internal Family Systems Model

Dr. Richard Schwartz developed Internal Family Systems (IFS) after noticing something his clients kept describing: They didn't feel like a unified self. They felt like a committee of different voices, different impulses, different versions of themselves (Schwartz, 1995).

Here's the core idea: **You have a Self, and you have Parts.**

Your **Self** is your essential core—calm, curious, compassionate, clear, connected. It's the part of you that can hold complexity, feel empathy, and make wise decisions. It's not damaged by trauma. It's always there, even when you can't access it.

Your **Parts** are the different strategies, roles, and protective mechanisms you developed to survive. They formed at different times, in response to different threats or pain. Each one has a positive intention—to protect you, keep you safe, help you survive.

The problem is, your parts don't always agree with each other. They don't coordinate. They fight for control. And most of them don't trust your Self to actually lead.

Think of it like this: You're supposed to be the calm, compassionate leader of your internal family. But instead, your parts have staged a coup. Some of them are running the show, making decisions based on old threats that no longer exist. Others are locked in the basement, holding pain you don't want to feel. And your Self—the one who should be in charge—can't get a word in.

This is what's happening when you do things you don't want to do, when you react in ways you regret, when you can't access the person you want to be.

Your parts are running the show. Your Self is sidelined.

The Three Types of Parts

In IFS, parts fall into three main categories: Exiles, Managers, and Firefighters. Let's break them down.

Exiles: The Wounded Ones

Exiles are the parts of you that hold the pain, shame, fear, and vulnerability from the past—especially from childhood.

These are the parts that experienced the trauma, the neglect, the rejection, the fear. They're often stuck in time, frozen at the age when the wounding happened. They hold the feelings that were too overwhelming to process at the time.

Your Exiles might be:

- The child who felt unloved and unworthy

- The teenager who was humiliated or rejected

- The part that holds terror from abuse

- The part that carries shame about who you are

Exiles are called exiles because your system has locked them away. They're too painful, too intense, too disruptive. If they came fully to the surface, you'd be overwhelmed. So your other parts work hard to keep them hidden.

But Exiles don't stay quiet forever. They leak out in unexpected ways—sudden waves of shame, unexplained terror, tears you don't understand, or reactions that seem way out of proportion to the situation.

Managers: The Protectors

Managers are the parts that try to keep your life under control so your Exiles never get triggered in the first place.

They're proactive protectors. They run your life, manage your relationships, control your environment. Their whole job is to prevent anything that might activate your Exiles' pain.

Common Manager strategies include:

Perfectionism: If everything is perfect, no one can criticize you. Criticism might trigger the Exile that feels worthless, so your Manager makes sure you never give anyone a reason to criticize you.

People-pleasing: If everyone likes you, no one will reject you. Rejection might trigger the Exile that felt abandoned, so your Manager makes sure you're always agreeable, always helpful, never a burden.

Intellectualizing: If you stay in your head, you don't have to feel your feelings. Feelings might connect you to your Exiles' pain, so your Manager keeps you analyzing, thinking, problem-solving— anything but feeling.

Hypervigilance: If you're always scanning for danger, you can prevent bad things before they happen. Your Manager learned that danger was always coming, so it never lets you relax.

Over-functioning: If you're always busy and productive, you don't have time to feel lonely or empty. Your Manager keeps you moving so you don't have to sit still with those uncomfortable feelings.

Managers aren't bad. They're actually trying to help. But they're exhausting. They run your life with an iron fist, never letting you rest, never letting you be spontaneous or vulnerable.

And here's the thing: **The harder your Managers work, the more desperate your Exiles become.** Your Exiles just want to be seen, to be heard, to be healed. But your Managers are terrified of that. So they double down on control.

Firefighters: The Rescuers

Firefighters are the emergency response team. They jump in when your Managers fail and an Exile gets triggered anyway.

While Managers are proactive, Firefighters are reactive. They show up after the pain has surfaced, and their job is to make it stop—immediately, by any means necessary.

Common Firefighter strategies include:

Dissociation: You disconnect from your body, from the moment, from yourself. You're there but not really there. This is your system's instant eject button.

Numbing behaviors: Binge-eating, excessive screen time, scrolling social media for hours, binge-watching shows—anything that distracts you from feeling.

Substance use: Alcohol, drugs, even excessive caffeine or sugar. Anything that changes your state quickly.

Rage or aggression: Anger can shut down vulnerability fast. If you're furious, you don't have to feel sad or scared.

Self-harm or risky behaviors: Sometimes Firefighters create a different kind of pain to distract from emotional pain. Or they create drama and crisis to pull focus.

Sexual behavior: Compulsive sexual activity or casual hookups that help you avoid intimacy or difficult feelings.

Firefighters get a bad rap. They're usually the parts people feel most ashamed of. But remember: **They're trying to help.** They're doing what they think they need to do to protect you from overwhelming pain.

The problem is, their solutions create new problems. They stop the pain temporarily, but they don't heal it. And often, their strategies harm you in other ways.

The Self: Your Compassionate Core

Underneath all these parts is your Self.

Your Self is different from your parts. It's not a role or a strategy. It's your essence—the calm, connected, clear presence that can lead your system.

When you're in Self, you feel the "8 C's" that Schwartz describes (Schwartz & Sweezy, 2020):

- **Calm:** Peaceful, not reactive

- **Curious:** Interested, wanting to understand

- **Clear:** Able to see situations accurately

- **Compassionate:** Feeling care for yourself and others

- **Confident:** Trusting your ability to handle things

- **Creative:** Able to think flexibly and find new solutions

- **Courageous:** Willing to face difficulty

- **Connected:** Feeling part of something larger than yourself

Sound familiar? This is the same as the ventral vagal state from Polyvagal Theory. Your Self *is* your Compassionate Core. It emerges when your nervous system feels safe.

The goal of healing isn't to get rid of parts. It's to help your Self become the leader of your internal system. When your Self is in charge, your parts can relax. They can trust that someone wise is running things. They don't have to protect you so desperately.

But this only happens when your parts believe your Self can actually handle what comes up. And they only believe that when they feel safe—which brings us back to the nervous system.

How Parts and States Interact

Here's where Polyvagal Theory and IFS come together beautifully:

When you're in a threat state (sympathetic or dorsal), your parts are in charge.

If your nervous system is activated (sympathetic), your Managers go into overdrive and your Firefighters are on standby. If your nervous system shuts down (dorsal), you can't access your parts at all— you're too numb to feel them.

When you're in a safe state (ventral), you can access your Self.

Only when your body feels genuinely safe can you access the calm, curious, compassionate presence of Self. This is when you can actually work with your parts.

This is why you can't "just be more compassionate" with yourself when you're activated. Your Manager parts won't let you. They're too busy trying to control everything. Or your system is too shut down to feel anything.

You need body regulation to access Self. And you need Self to heal your parts.

They work together. They're not separate processes—they're two sides of the same coin.

Jennifer's Story: Meeting Her Parts

Jennifer, a 29-year-old teacher, came to therapy because she couldn't maintain relationships. Every time someone got close, she'd push them away or sabotage things.

"I want connection," she'd say. "But when someone actually cares about me, I panic. I find reasons they're wrong for me. Or I pick fights until they leave."

When she learned about parts, she started to see her pattern clearly.

She had an Exile—a young part that felt deeply unlovable. This part got formed when her father left when she was six and her mother emotionally checked out after that. The message this part internalized: "People you love leave. You're not worth staying for."

To protect this Exile, Jennifer developed a Manager that she called "The Skeptic." This part evaluated every potential relationship and found flaws. It kept her at a distance. Its logic: "If I don't let anyone close, they can't leave me."

But sometimes someone would slip through The Skeptic's defenses. Someone would be persistent, genuine, kind. Jennifer would start to feel hope. She'd let herself be vulnerable.

And then a Firefighter would kick in—Jennifer called it "The Saboteur." This part would create fights, withdraw suddenly, or find reasons to end things. Its logic: "Get out before they leave. Leave first. Don't give them the chance to hurt you."

Jennifer could see this pattern intellectually. But she couldn't stop it. Why?

Because she was trying to work with her parts while her nervous system was dysregulated. Every time a relationship triggered her Exile's fear, her system would activate (sympathetic) or shut down

35

(dorsal). In those states, her protective parts (The Skeptic, The Saboteur) ran the show.

The breakthrough came when she learned to regulate her nervous system first. When she felt that panic rising, instead of listening to The Skeptic or acting on The Saboteur's impulses, she'd pause. She'd use her anchoring practices (we'll cover these in the next section) to get her body back to a place of safety.

Then, from that calm, connected state—from Self—she could talk to her parts. She could thank The Skeptic for trying to protect her. She could understand that The Saboteur was actually trying to help, in its desperate way.

And slowly, she could make space for that young Exile to be seen, to tell its story, to learn that Jennifer was no longer six years old and powerless.

This didn't happen overnight. But it did happen. And it started with understanding that her parts weren't the problem. They were just doing their jobs. The problem was that nobody was leading—her Self needed to step into that role.

The Worksheet: Identifying Your Key Players

Let's get specific about your parts.

You probably have dozens of parts, but let's start with the ones that show up most often—your most active Managers and Firefighters.

Identifying Your Managers:

Managers are the parts that run your daily life. They're the strategies you use all the time to feel safe, in control, worthy.

Ask yourself:

1. **What do I do to try to control my life or prevent bad things from happening?** (Examples: planning excessively, people-pleasing, perfectionism, staying busy, hypervigilance)

36

2. **What would I be terrified might happen if I stopped doing these things?** (This tells you what your Manager is protecting you from)

3. **What rules or beliefs guide my behavior?** (Examples: "If I'm not perfect, I'm worthless." "If I say no, people will abandon me." "If I relax, something bad will happen.")

Write down your top 2-3 Manager parts. Give them names if you want—it makes them easier to work with. "The Perfectionist." "The People-Pleaser." "The Critic."

Identifying Your Firefighters:

Firefighters are reactive. They show up when you're already in pain or when an Exile has been triggered.

Ask yourself:

1. **When I'm overwhelmed or in emotional pain, what do I do to make it stop?** (Examples: dissociate, binge-eat, scroll social media for hours, drink, pick fights, engage in risky behavior)

2. **What behaviors do I feel ashamed of but keep doing anyway?** (Firefighters often operate in ways we later regret)

3. **What do these behaviors help me avoid feeling?** (This tells you what pain your Firefighter is trying to protect you from)

Write down your top 2-3 Firefighter parts.

Identifying Your Exiles (Gently):

You don't need to fully access your Exiles yet—we'll do that carefully in later chapters. For now, just see if you can sense them.

Ask yourself:

1. **What feelings come up that feel overwhelming or intolerable?** (Shame, worthlessness, terror, abandonment, etc.)

2. **When those feelings start to surface, what do you notice?** (Do your Managers immediately try to distract you? Do your Firefighters kick in to numb you out?)

3. **If you imagine a younger version of yourself who holds those feelings, how old are they? What are they experiencing?**

Just notice. Don't force anything. If you feel nothing, that's okay— you might be in a dorsal shutdown state or your protectors are working hard to keep Exiles hidden. We'll work with that.

The Most Important Question:

Who's leading your system most of the time—your Self or your parts?

When you make decisions, is it from a place of calm wisdom (Self)? Or is it from anxiety, control, fear, or numbness (parts)?

There's no judgment here. Most trauma survivors are led by their parts most of the time. That's the starting point. Now you know what needs to change.

Why This Changes Everything

Once you start seeing your parts, your whole experience shifts.

Instead of "I am anxious," you think "My Manager is activated right now."

Instead of "I'm such a mess, I can't stop binge-eating," you think "My Firefighter is trying to help me avoid some pain. What's it protecting me from?"

Instead of "Why can't I just get over this?" you think "My Exile is still hurting and my protectors won't let me near it because they don't trust that I can handle it."

This isn't just reframing. This is fundamentally changing your relationship with yourself.

You're not broken. You're not a mess. You're a Self with parts that are doing their absolute best to protect you, using outdated strategies that once worked but now don't.

Your job isn't to get rid of parts or suppress them or fight them. Your job is to lead them—to help them update their understanding of what you need, to help them trust that you (your Self) can handle things, to give them permission to rest.

But you can only do that from Self. And you can only access Self when your nervous system is regulated.

Which is why, in the next chapter, we're going to address the core problem that keeps you stuck: trying to work with your parts when your body is in survival mode.

What Matters Most

You're not a single, unified self. You're a healthy Self with multiple parts, each playing different roles to keep you safe. You have Exiles that hold pain from the past, Managers that try to prevent that pain from surfacing, and Firefighters that react when the pain breaks through anyway. None of these parts are bad—they're all trying to help you survive.

Your Self is your calm, compassionate core—the part of you that can lead your internal system with wisdom and care. It's not damaged by trauma and it's always there, but you can't access it when your nervous system is in a threat state. When you're anxious or shut down, your protective parts run the show, not your Self.

Healing isn't about eliminating your parts or fighting against them. It's about helping your Self become the leader of your internal system so your parts can finally relax. They've been running things because they didn't trust anyone else could handle the job. Your task is to show them, gradually and consistently, that your Self is capable of leading.

Chapter 4: The Core Problem: Why You Can't "Just Talk" to Your Trauma

Let's talk about why therapy doesn't always work.

Not because therapists are bad at their jobs. Not because you're "resistant to treatment." But because there's a fundamental misunderstanding about how trauma healing actually works.

Traditional talk therapy was built on the idea that insight leads to change. Understand your problems, make connections between past and present, reframe your thinking, and you'll feel better.

For many issues, this works great. For complex trauma, it doesn't.

Because here's the thing nobody explained to you: **You can't heal your parts when your nervous system is in survival mode.**

This is the core problem. This is why you've read all the books, done all the exercises, understood all the patterns—and still feel stuck.

You've been trying to do mind-work while your body is screaming that you're in danger.

The Integration Disconnect

Remember the two systems we've been exploring:

Polyvagal Theory explains your nervous system states. You need to be in ventral vagal (safe and social) to access healing.

Internal Family Systems explains your parts. You need to be in Self to lead your system with compassion.

Here's the key insight: **Self and ventral vagal are the same state.**

When your nervous system is regulated, you can access Self. When you're in Self, your nervous system is regulated. They're two descriptions of the same experience—one from a body perspective (Polyvagal), one from a psychological perspective (IFS).

Your Compassionate Core exists at the intersection of these two.

The problem:

When you're in sympathetic activation (fight-or-flight), you can't access Self. Your Manager parts are running the show. They're in control mode, trying desperately to keep you safe. They're not going to step aside and let you explore painful feelings or access vulnerability. That feels dangerous to them.

When you're in dorsal shutdown (freeze/collapse), you can't feel your parts at all. You're numb, disconnected, foggy. There's no access to Self, no access to Exiles, no access to anything. You're just... gone.

Only when you're in ventral vagal safety can you access the Self that can actually work with your parts.

This is the Golden Rule of trauma integration: **Regulate the body first, then work with the parts.**

Why Traditional Therapy Often Fails

Think about a typical therapy session for trauma.

You sit down. Your therapist asks you to talk about what happened. You start describing a painful memory or difficult experience.

What happens in your body?

If you're like most trauma survivors, one of two things:

Option 1: You activate.

Your heart starts racing. Your breathing gets shallow. You feel anxious, maybe panicky. You start thinking about it too much, intellectualizing, explaining, defending. Your thoughts spiral.

This is sympathetic activation. Your nervous system perceives the memory as a current threat. It's mobilizing you to fight or flee— except there's nothing to fight or flee from. You're just sitting in a chair, talking.

In this state, you can't access Self. Your Manager parts have jumped in to protect you. Maybe The Critic starts judging you: "This is stupid. It wasn't that bad. Stop being dramatic." Maybe The Analyzer starts overexplaining: "Let me tell you exactly why this happened and what it means." Maybe The Defender gets activated: "Actually, it wasn't their fault because..."

You're not in Self. You're in protection mode. And from protection mode, you can't actually heal.

Option 2: You shut down.

You go numb. You feel disconnected, like you're describing someone else's life. You can say the words, but you don't feel anything. Maybe you dissociate—you're looking at yourself from outside, or time feels weird, or you just space out entirely.

This is dorsal shutdown. Your nervous system has decided this is too much, so it's hit the circuit breaker. You're immobilized, offline.

In this state, you also can't access Self. You can't feel your parts. You can't access compassion or curiosity. You're just surviving the moment, waiting for it to be over.

In either state, healing doesn't happen.

You're not processing the trauma. You're either defending against it (sympathetic) or dissociating from it (dorsal). You might gain some intellectual understanding. You might feel a bit better because you've "talked about it." But the trauma isn't actually integrating. Your nervous system hasn't learned that you're safe. Your Exiles haven't been witnessed. Your protective parts haven't been reassured.

The "Just Feel Your Feelings" Trap

43

You've probably heard this advice: "Just sit with your feelings. Let yourself feel them."

Sounds reasonable, right? Trauma survivors avoid feelings because feelings are overwhelming, so obviously you need to learn to feel them.

Except that advice misses something crucial: **Your protective parts won't let you feel overwhelming feelings because they're trying to keep you safe.**

When you try to "just feel" pain that an Exile is holding, your Managers and Firefighters immediately jump in. They're not being difficult. They're doing their job. They learned a long time ago that those feelings are dangerous—they're associated with real threats, real helplessness, real trauma.

So when you try to force yourself to feel, one of several things happens:

1. **Your Managers shut it down.** You suddenly can't access the feeling. You go blank. You start thinking instead of feeling. You minimize it.

2. **Your Firefighters react.** You get overwhelmed and immediately reach for numbing behaviors—food, screens, substance use, dissociation.

3. **You flood.** You drop into the feeling so completely that you're no longer present. You're not "with" the feeling as your Self—you're *in* it, reliving it, overwhelmed by it.

None of these are healing. The first two are avoidance. The third is retraumatization.

Real healing happens when you can be with a feeling from Self—present, curious, compassionate, not overwhelmed.

And you can only do that when your nervous system is regulated enough to access Self in the first place.

The Sequence That Actually Works

Here's the sequence for trauma integration that honors both your body and your parts:

Step 1: Regulate your nervous system.

Before you do anything else, before you try to access feelings or work with parts, you need to get your body to a place of relative safety. Not perfectly calm—that's not realistic. But enough ventral vagal activation that you can think clearly, feel connected to yourself, access some curiosity and compassion.

This might take 5 minutes. It might take 30 minutes. It might take practicing all day, every day, for weeks before you can reliably access this state.

That's okay. This is the foundation. Without it, nothing else works.

Step 2: Connect with Self.

Once your body is relatively calm, check: Are you in Self? Do you feel curious about what's happening? Can you access compassion for yourself? Does your inner experience feel spacious rather than pressured?

If not, go back to Step 1. Your nervous system isn't regulated enough yet, or your Manager parts are still running the show.

If yes, continue.

Step 3: Work with your protector parts first.

Don't go straight for the pain. Don't try to access your Exiles yet.

First, talk to the parts that are protecting you—your Managers and Firefighters. Thank them for their work. Get curious about what

45

they're afraid would happen if they stepped aside. Reassure them that you (your Self) can handle what comes up.

This step is essential. If your protectors don't trust you, they won't let you near your Exiles. And forcing past them just makes them more desperate and rigid.

Step 4: Once your protectors give permission, gently witness your Exiles.

Only now, when your body is regulated AND your protectors trust you, can you safely access the wounded parts that hold the trauma.

And even then, you go slowly. You stay in Self. You don't merge with the Exile's feelings—you witness them. You're with the part, not consumed by it.

This is the healing moment: An Exile finally being seen, heard, and held by a compassionate presence (your Self) who isn't overwhelmed, isn't trying to fix it, isn't rejecting it. Just being with it.

This sequence can't be rushed. And you can't skip steps.

If you try to access your Exiles before your protectors are ready, your protectors will sabotage the process. If you try to work with any parts before your nervous system is regulated, you won't have access to Self, and it won't be healing—it'll just be parts talking to parts.

David's Story: The Stuck Cycle

David, a 37-year-old software engineer, had been in therapy on and off for a decade. He understood his trauma intellectually. He could explain exactly how his childhood abuse affected him. He knew his patterns.

But nothing changed.

"I've talked about it so many times," he said. "I'm tired of talking about it. I know the story. I know why I am the way I am. So why doesn't it get better?"

What David didn't know was that every time he talked about his trauma in therapy, he was either activating his nervous system (going into hyperanalysis, intellectualizing, explaining) or shutting down (dissociating, feeling nothing).

He'd describe a memory, and his therapist would say, "How does that make you feel?" And David would either launch into a cognitive analysis or say, "I don't know. I don't really feel anything."

He wasn't being resistant. He wasn't "not trying." His nervous system was doing exactly what it was trained to do—either mobilize to analyze the threat or shut down to avoid overwhelm.

His protective parts (particularly a strong Manager that David called "The Analyst") would not let him actually feel the pain. Why? Because they didn't trust that David could handle it without falling apart.

The breakthrough came when David learned the sequence.

First, he practiced regulating his nervous system—finding his ventral vagal anchor, learning what safety felt like in his body. This took weeks. He wasn't trying to process trauma yet. He was just building the capacity to be present and calm.

Then, he started getting to know his protectors. He'd talk to The Analyst: "What are you afraid would happen if I actually felt my feelings about this?" The Analyst's answer: "You'd fall apart. You'd be weak. You'd be vulnerable like you were as a kid, and that's dangerous."

David (from Self) could reassure The Analyst: "I'm not a kid anymore. I'm an adult. I can handle these feelings. I won't fall apart. But I need you to step aside a little so I can actually process this."

This wasn't one conversation. It was dozens of conversations, building trust over time.

Eventually, The Analyst relaxed enough to let David access the younger Exile that held the fear and pain from childhood. And because David's nervous system was regulated and his Self was leading, he could finally witness that part's pain without either intellectualizing it away or being overwhelmed by it.

That's when healing happened. Not when he talked about the trauma. Not when he understood it. But when he could be present with the wounded part of himself from a place of grounded, compassionate connection.

When You're in Shutdown, You Can't Feel Your Parts

There's a special challenge with dorsal shutdown that needs addressing.

When you're in sympathetic activation, your protector parts are very active—you can feel them. The anxiety, the hypervigilance, the inner critic, the people-pleasing. They're loud.

But when you're in dorsal shutdown, you can't feel anything.

This is why people in chronic shutdown often say, "I don't have parts. I don't feel conflicted. I just feel nothing."

They do have parts. But they're not accessible because the nervous system is offline. Trying to do parts work from dorsal shutdown is like trying to use a computer that's been unplugged. The programs are there—they're just not running.

If you're in shutdown, your first job is to gently mobilize your system—to climb back up the ladder from dorsal to sympathetic to ventral. This might mean moving your body, connecting with others, engaging with the world in small ways.

Only once you have some activation (without being overwhelmed) can you start accessing and working with parts.

When You're Activated, Your Protectors Are in Charge

If you're in sympathetic activation, your protective parts (usually Managers) are running the show.

In this state, they're not interested in healing. They're interested in control. They want to analyze, fix, explain, defend, perfect, achieve—anything that gives them a sense of managing the threat they perceive.

Trying to access your Exiles from this state is like trying to have a deep, vulnerable conversation while someone is honking a car horn in your face. Your protectors won't allow it. It's not the right time.

First, you need to regulate. Then, you need to negotiate with your protectors—to help them understand that you're safe enough now to do this work.

Then, and only then, can you access the vulnerable parts that need healing.

The Golden Rule: Regulate First

This is the most important thing in this entire book:

You cannot heal your mind's parts until you can regulate your body's state.

Say it again. Write it down. Tattoo it somewhere.

Every time you try to do trauma work and it doesn't work, check: What state is my nervous system in? Am I trying to do Self-led healing when I'm actually in a protector-led survival state?

If you're activated or shut down, stop. Don't push through. Don't force it. Just come back to regulating your nervous system. Find your anchor. Get back to ventral.

Then try again.

This isn't a sign of weakness. This is honoring how your system actually works.

What This Means Going Forward

The rest of this book follows the sequence we've just described.

The next section (Part 2) gives you the practical tools to work with your nervous system and your parts—in the right order.

You'll learn how to find your ventral vagal anchor (Step 1).

You'll learn how to work with your Manager parts (Step 2) and your Firefighter parts (Step 3).

You'll learn how to safely witness your Exiles (Step 4).

And you'll learn how to integrate all of this into your daily life (Step 5).

But it all starts with understanding this core principle: **Regulation first. Then transformation.**

Your body has to feel safe before your mind can heal.

That's not a bug in the system. That's how it's designed.

The Bottom Line

You can't access your Self when your nervous system is in a threat state. When you're anxious and activated, your protective Manager parts are in control, refusing to let you near vulnerable feelings. When you're numb and shut down, you can't feel your parts at all. Only when your body is in a state of relative safety can you access the calm, compassionate presence that can actually heal.

This is why traditional talk therapy often fails with complex trauma. You sit down to process painful memories, but your nervous system either activates in defense or shuts down in protection. In either state, real healing can't happen. You're either fighting the feelings or disconnected from them, never actually present with them in a way that allows integration.

The sequence that works is non-negotiable: regulate your nervous system first, connect with your Self, work with your protector parts to build trust, and only then gently witness your wounded Exiles. This isn't about understanding your trauma intellectually. It's about creating the physiological safety that allows your parts to finally trust that healing is possible without falling apart.

Chapter 5: Find Your "Ventral Vagal" Anchor

Here's the problem with most advice about calming down: It doesn't work.

"Just breathe." "Try to relax." "Don't worry about it." These phrases are useless when your nervous system is convinced you're in danger. It's like telling someone who's drowning to "just swim better."

When your body is in sympathetic activation or dorsal shutdown, conscious commands to "calm down" don't reach the part of your nervous system that's running the show. Your autonomic nervous system operates below conscious awareness. Willpower can't override it.

So what does work?

You need to give your nervous system *somatic* experiences—body-based cues—that genuinely signal safety. Not intellectual concepts of safety. Not logical reassurance. Actual, physical, felt experiences that your nervous system recognizes as "You're okay right now."

This is what I call finding your **ventral vagal anchor.**

Your anchor is the felt sense of safety in your body. It's that rare moment when your shoulders drop, your breathing eases, and you feel... okay. Present. Connected. Yourself.

For most trauma survivors, this state is brief and infrequent. But it exists. And once you learn to recognize it, you can learn to access it more often.

This chapter teaches you how.

The Concept of "Glimmers"

Before we talk about finding safety, let's talk about what safety actually feels like.

Trauma survivors are experts at noticing threats. You've been trained to scan for danger, to spot the warning signs, to prepare for the worst. This is *neuroception* working overtime—your nervous system's constant surveillance for cues of danger (Porges, 2011).

You know what triggers feel like. The tightness in your chest when someone raises their voice. The pit in your stomach when plans change unexpectedly. The fog that descends when emotions get too big.

But can you identify what safety feels like?

Deb Dana, a clinician who applies Polyvagal Theory in therapy, coined the term **"glimmers"** to describe the opposite of triggers (Dana, 2018). Glimmers are small moments when your nervous system registers safety, connection, or ease—even briefly.

A glimmer might be:

- The warmth of sun on your face
- Your dog greeting you at the door
- The first sip of coffee in the morning
- A genuine smile from a stranger
- The relief of finishing a task
- Music that makes you feel something
- The weight of a blanket
- A moment of eye contact with someone you trust

These aren't big, dramatic experiences. They're micro-moments. Most people miss them entirely because they're scanning for threats, not for safety.

But your nervous system notices glimmers, even when you don't. And when you start paying attention to them, you can use them intentionally.

Why Glimmers Matter

Here's what most people don't understand about nervous system regulation: **You can't just "stop" being anxious or numb. You have to give your system something else to move toward.**

Your nervous system is always in a state. Sympathetic, dorsal, or ventral. It doesn't just turn off.

When you try to force yourself to calm down from sympathetic activation, you're essentially trying to push your system from mobilization to stillness. That often backfires—your system resists because it's convinced the mobilization is necessary.

But when you give your system a glimmer—a genuine cue of safety—you're offering it a pathway toward ventral. You're not forcing anything. You're inviting your nervous system to notice: "Oh, actually, there's safety here. I can shift."

This is why deep breathing sometimes works and sometimes doesn't. If you're using breath as a command ("Calm down NOW"), your system resists. If you're using breath as an invitation ("Here's a cue of safety you can notice"), your system might accept.

Building Your Glimmer Practice

Start noticing glimmers in your daily life.

Don't try to create them yet. Just notice when they happen naturally.

Throughout your day, when you feel even a slight sense of ease or okayness—even for two seconds—pause. Notice it. Name it.

"There's a glimmer. I feel a bit lighter right now."

That's it. You don't need to hold onto it. You don't need to make it last. Just notice it when it's there.

Some people find it helpful to keep a glimmer journal for a week. At the end of each day, write down 1-3 moments when you felt any degree of safety, calm, or connection. They'll be small. That's fine. Small is what we're looking for.

What you're doing is training your attention. Your nervous system has been trained to notice danger. Now you're teaching it to notice safety too.

Somatic Anchors: Direct Pathways to Safety

Glimmers happen naturally. But you can also create them deliberately through specific somatic practices—body-based techniques that directly activate your ventral vagal system.

These aren't relaxation techniques in the traditional sense. They're not about "trying to calm down." They're about giving your nervous system specific physiological inputs that it recognizes as safety signals.

Let's look at the most effective ones.

The Vagal Sigh

This is one of the simplest and most effective techniques for shifting your nervous system state.

A vagal sigh is a specific breathing pattern that activates your vagus nerve—the main nerve of your parasympathetic system (Balban et al., 2023). It's not regular deep breathing. It has a unique pattern:

How to do it:

1. Inhale through your nose—a normal breath, not too deep

2. At the top of that inhale, take another small sip of air (a mini-inhale on top of the first one)

3. Exhale slowly through your mouth with a sigh

The key is the double inhale. That's what maximally expands your lungs and triggers the vagal response.

Do this 2-3 times in a row.

You should feel a subtle shift—maybe your shoulders drop, or your jaw unclenches, or your thoughts slow down just a bit. That's your system moving toward ventral.

When to use it: Anytime you notice sympathetic activation. Racing thoughts, tight chest, shallow breathing, rising anxiety. The vagal sigh can interrupt the activation and give your system a reset point.

Grounding Through Your Feet

When you're anxious or dissociated, you're disconnected from your body and your present environment. Grounding brings you back.

How to do it:

1. Stand or sit with your feet flat on the floor

2. Notice the sensation of your feet touching the ground—the pressure, the texture, the temperature

3. Press your feet gently but firmly into the floor

4. Notice how the ground supports you. You don't have to hold yourself up—the ground is doing that

5. Stay with this sensation for 30-60 seconds

When to use it: When you're spinning in your head, when you're dissociating, when you feel unmoored or overwhelmed. This practice brings you back to your body and the present moment.

Sensory Orientation

Your eyes are directly connected to your nervous system. When you're in threat, your vision narrows—you focus intensely on the perceived danger. When you're safe, your vision softens and widens.

You can use your vision intentionally to signal safety to your nervous system.

How to do it:

1. Without moving your head, let your eyes wander slowly around your environment

2. Notice colors, shapes, textures—just observe without analyzing

3. Let your gaze settle on something pleasant or neutral—a plant, a piece of art, the sky outside

4. Soften your focus. Instead of staring intently, let your vision be gentle and wide

5. Take in your peripheral vision—what do you notice on the edges of your sight?

This technique is called "orienting" because you're orienting to your actual, present environment rather than the threat your nervous system is imagining (Levine, 1997).

When to use it: When you're in hypervigilance mode, when your thoughts are catastrophizing, when you feel like danger is everywhere. This reminds your system: "Look around. Right here, right now, you're okay."

The Hand on Heart Practice

Physical touch can be deeply regulating, especially self-touch. This practice uses gentle pressure and warmth to activate your ventral system.

How to do it:

1. Place one or both hands on your heart center (your chest)

2. Apply gentle, warm pressure

3. Feel the warmth from your hands, the rise and fall of your breath, the beating of your heart

4. You might silently say something compassionate to yourself: "I'm here." "It's okay." "I've got you."

This practice combines physical grounding with self-compassion. It's simple but surprisingly powerful (Neff & Germer, 2018).

When to use it: When you're feeling scared, alone, or overwhelmed. When you need to feel connected to yourself. When your inner critic is loud and you need to access Self.

Humming or Singing

Your vagus nerve runs through your vocal cords. When you make sounds—especially humming or singing—you're literally vibrating your vagus nerve, which activates your parasympathetic system (Porges, 2017).

How to do it:

1. Hum any note that feels comfortable—low or high, doesn't matter

2. Feel the vibration in your throat and chest

3. Hum for 30-60 seconds

4. Or, if you prefer, sing—it doesn't have to be good, just has to be done

When to use it: When you're feeling shut down (dorsal) and need to gently mobilize your system. When you're alone and need a quick nervous system shift. When you're overwhelmed and need to create a different sensation in your body.

Cold Exposure

Brief exposure to cold water can interrupt a sympathetic spiral and create a physiological shift.

How to do it:

1. Splash cold water on your face, or

2. Hold an ice cube in your hand, or

3. Take a brief cold shower

The cold triggers something called the "dive reflex"—an automatic response that slows your heart rate and shifts your nervous system (Khurana et al., 1980).

When to use it: When you're in intense panic or rage (high sympathetic activation) and nothing else is working. This is a circuit-breaker technique—it creates such a strong physical sensation that your system has to respond.

Caution: This one is intense. Don't use it if you're already in dorsal shutdown—it could push you further down. Only use it for high activation.

Movement and Shaking

Sometimes your body needs to move to complete the stress cycle. Trauma can get stuck as incomplete fight-or-flight responses—your body mobilized for action but couldn't act (Levine, 1997).

How to do it:

1. Shake out your hands vigorously for 30 seconds

2. Shake your whole body—arms, legs, torso—like you're shaking off water

3. Or go for a brief, brisk walk

4. Or do jumping jacks, dance, or any movement that feels good

This releases held tension and helps your system complete the activation cycle.

When to use it: When you're restless, agitated, or your body feels tight and coiled. When you have nervous energy with nowhere to go. When you've been sitting with difficult emotions and need to move.

Creating Your Personal Anchor Menu

Here's the practical part: You need a menu of 1-minute practices you can use anytime.

Not everything works for everyone. You need to find what works for your nervous system. And what works might change depending on what state you're in.

The Exercise: Build Your Anchor Menu

Over the next week, try each of the practices above. Notice what happens in your body when you do them.

For each practice, ask yourself:

- Does this help me feel more present?

- Does my breathing ease at all?

- Do I feel any shift toward calm or connection?

- Does this make things worse (more activated or more shut down)?

Based on your observations, create three lists:

List 1: For Sympathetic Activation (anxiety, panic, agitation)
Which practices help when you're anxious or wound up?

Maybe: Vagal sigh, grounding through feet, sensory orientation, cold exposure

List 2: For Dorsal Shutdown (numbness, fog, dissociation)
Which practices help when you're numb or checked out?

Maybe: Movement and shaking, humming, grounding through feet, cold exposure (gentle)

List 3: For General Regulation (building ventral capacity)
Which practices feel good when you're already relatively calm and you want to strengthen your ventral state?

Maybe: Hand on heart, humming, sensory orientation, noticing glimmers

Write these lists down. Keep them in your phone. These are your anchors—your reliable pathways back to your Compassionate Core.

Rachel's Story: Finding Her Anchors

Rachel, a 32-year-old nurse, lived in constant sympathetic activation. Work was stressful, her relationships were tense, and she couldn't remember the last time she felt truly relaxed.

When she learned about nervous system states, she started tracking hers. Turns out, she spent about 90% of her waking hours activated—heart racing, jaw clenched, mind spinning.

The remaining 10%? Dorsal shutdown. Collapsing on the couch, scrolling her phone, feeling nothing. Zero middle ground. No ventral time.

She tried the anchoring practices. Some worked immediately. Some didn't.

What worked for Rachel:

The vagal sigh was instant relief. Two breaths and she could feel her system downshift. She started using it dozens of times a day— before entering a patient's room, after a difficult conversation, in traffic.

Grounding through her feet worked when she felt scattered. At work, she'd take 30 seconds to stand, press her feet into the floor, and orient to her body. It brought her back when she felt like she was spinning.

What *didn't* work: Hand on heart made her feel more vulnerable and activated her protector parts. Cold exposure felt too intense. Humming felt silly.

That's fine. She didn't need every technique. She needed 2-3 reliable ones.

Over time, she built more capacity. She started noticing glimmers—moments when she actually felt okay. The smile from a patient's family member. The taste of her morning tea. The moment she sat down after a long shift.

She couldn't hold these states long. But she could find them. And finding them more often started to build a new pathway in her nervous system—a pathway to safety.

The Practice: Stacking Glimmers

Once you can notice glimmers and use somatic anchors, you can start stacking them—deliberately moving from one small experience of safety to another, building your ventral capacity.

Here's how it works:

1. Notice a glimmer or create one with an anchor practice

2. Stay with that sensation for 10-20 seconds. Don't rush past it.

3. Really notice what safety feels like in your body—even if it's subtle

4. Then find another glimmer or use another anchor

5. Notice that sensation for 10-20 seconds

6. Continue for 2-3 minutes

You're not trying to force a permanent state change. You're giving your nervous system repeated micro-doses of safety. Over time, these add up.

Think of it like exercise. One bicep curl doesn't build muscle. But doing it consistently over time does. Same with ventral regulation.

What This Isn't

This isn't about toxic positivity. You're not ignoring real problems or pretending everything is fine when it isn't.

You're also not "just relaxing" or "treating yourself." Those concepts miss the point entirely.

What you're doing is retraining your autonomic nervous system. You're creating new neural pathways. You're teaching your body that safety is possible, that calm is accessible, that you can return to your Compassionate Core even after you've been knocked out of it.

This is neurophysiological work. It's changing how your body responds to the world.

And it's foundational. Without this, the rest of the steps won't work.

Common Obstacles

"I can't feel anything."

If you're in chronic dorsal shutdown, you might not feel much when you try these practices. That's okay. You're still having an effect, even if you can't sense it yet. Keep practicing. Sensation will return gradually.

"I feel worse when I try to calm down."

This happens when your protector parts perceive calm as dangerous. They've learned that letting your guard down leads to bad things. We'll work with those parts in the next chapter. For now, try practices that feel neutral rather than explicitly calming.

"This feels fake or forced."

Your nervous system is skeptical. It's been in threat mode for a long time. Of course this feels strange. Keep going anyway. Over time, these states will feel less foreign.

"It works for a minute, then I'm anxious again."

That's normal. You're not aiming for permanent calm. You're building the muscle of returning to ventral. Each time you practice, you're strengthening that pathway.

Integration: Making This Real

Your anchor practices only work if you actually use them.

Here's how to integrate this into your daily life:

Set 3-5 reminders on your phone throughout the day. When the reminder goes off, pause for 60 seconds and use one anchor practice. Just one minute.

Link anchor practices to existing routines. Every morning when you pour your coffee, do a vagal sigh. Every time you sit in your car, ground through your feet. Every time you wash your hands, notice a glimmer.

Use anchors before transitions. Before a meeting, before a difficult conversation, before bed—anchor yourself first. This prepares your nervous system for what's ahead.

Use anchors after triggers. When you notice you've been activated or shut down, don't just push through. Pause. Anchor. Then continue.

The goal is to make these practices automatic—like brushing your teeth. Your nervous system needs consistent repetition to learn new patterns.

This Is Step One

Finding your anchor is the foundation for everything else in this book.

You can't work with your parts until your body feels safe. You can't access Self until you're in ventral. You can't heal your Exiles until your protectors trust that you can handle it.

All of that requires nervous system regulation first.

So practice. Build your anchor menu. Use it throughout your day. Get familiar with what ventral feels like in your body.

Then, once you can reliably find your Compassionate Core—even briefly—you're ready for the next step: working with your protector parts.

What You've Learned

Your nervous system needs somatic experiences of safety, not intellectual reassurance. Glimmers are micro-moments when your body registers ease, connection, or calm—the opposite of triggers. Most trauma survivors never notice glimmers because they're trained to scan for danger, but learning to recognize these moments trains your attention toward safety.

You can create glimmers deliberately through somatic anchors— practices like the vagal sigh, grounding through your feet, sensory orientation, and self-touch. These aren't relaxation techniques; they're direct physiological inputs that activate your ventral vagal system. Different practices work for different nervous system states, so you need to build a personalized menu of what actually shifts your system.

This is foundational work. Without the ability to access your Compassionate Core through nervous system regulation, you can't effectively work with your parts or heal your trauma. Practice your anchors daily, build your ventral capacity gradually, and recognize that each micro-dose of safety is creating new neural pathways that make regulation easier over time.

Chapter 6: Befriend Your Protectors (The Managers)

Your inner critic is not your enemy.

I know that sounds wrong. The voice in your head that tells you you're not good enough, that picks apart everything you do, that won't let you rest—how could that not be the enemy?

But here's what changes everything: **Your inner critic is a protector part trying desperately to keep you safe.**

It's not trying to hurt you. It's trying to prevent you from being hurt by others. It learned, probably long ago, that if you could just be perfect enough, controlled enough, smart enough, then maybe you'd be safe. Maybe you wouldn't be criticized, rejected, or hurt.

Your Manager parts—including that harsh inner critic—developed for a reason. They're not personality defects. They're strategies that once worked, or at least tried to work, to keep a younger, more vulnerable version of you from experiencing pain.

The problem is, they're still running strategies designed for old threats that no longer exist. And they won't stop until they trust that you (your Self) can actually handle your life without their rigid control.

This chapter teaches you how to work with your Managers—not by fighting them, but by befriending them.

Recognizing Your Managers in Action

Before you can work with your Managers, you need to recognize when they're active.

Most of the time, you don't notice them. They've been running your life for so long that their voice sounds like your own voice. Their strategies feel like "just how you are."

But Managers have tells. Once you know what to look for, you can spot them.

Your Managers are active when you:

- Feel compelled to be productive, even when you're exhausted

- Can't stop analyzing or intellectualizing a situation

- Obsess over small details or mistakes

- Feel anxious about other people's opinions of you

- Try to control outcomes or other people's behavior

- Push yourself to be perfect or excellent

- Avoid conflict at all costs

- Overexplain or justify your choices

- Feel guilty when you rest or do something just for enjoyment

- Scan constantly for what could go wrong

These are all Manager strategies. They're not you. They're parts of you, trying to manage your life in ways that once made sense.

The Shift: From Part to Self

The key skill you need to develop is **noticing when a Manager is driving versus when your Self is leading.**

When a Manager is driving, you feel pressured, controlled, anxious, or compulsive. There's no space, no choice. You *have* to do the thing the Manager wants you to do, or else.

When Self is leading, you feel calm, curious, and compassionate. There's space. You can see options. You can choose your response.

Here's a simple practice to build this awareness:

Throughout your day, when you notice you're in a Manager-driven state, say this to yourself:

"There's a part of me that's _____."

Fill in the blank with what the Manager is doing.

"There's a part of me that's criticizing my work."

"There's a part of me that's trying to control this situation."

"There's a part of me that's terrified of disappointing people."

Notice the language: "There's a **part** of me." Not "I am." This creates distance. This helps you see that you (Self) are not the Manager. You *have* a Manager part, but you're not it.

This tiny linguistic shift is powerful. It starts to separate Self from parts.

The Manager Dialogue Process

Once you can recognize a Manager is active, you can start working with it.

This is not about shutting it down or arguing with it. Managers get more rigid when you fight them. They dig in harder.

Instead, you're going to get curious. You're going to ask the Manager what it's trying to do for you.

But (and this is crucial) **you can only do this when you're anchored in your Compassionate Core.**

If you try to work with a Manager while you're in sympathetic activation or dorsal shutdown, you won't be in Self. You'll just have one part talking to another part. That doesn't create change.

So first, use your anchor practices. Get yourself into ventral. Access Self—that calm, curious, compassionate presence.

Then, try this:

The Four-Question Process

Question 1: "What are you trying to do for me right now?"

Ask the Manager directly. Listen for the answer. It might come as words, as images, as a felt sense.

Example: Your inner critic is harsh after you made a small mistake at work.

You (from Self): "Inner critic, what are you trying to do for me right now?"

Inner critic: "I'm trying to make you better. If I point out every mistake, maybe you won't make them again."

Question 2: "What are you afraid would happen if you stopped doing this?"

This is the key question. It reveals what the Manager is protecting you from.

You: "What are you afraid would happen if you stopped criticizing me?"

Inner critic: "If I don't criticize you, you'll get complacent. You'll mess up. People will judge you, reject you, see that you're not actually competent."

There it is. The Manager isn't trying to hurt you. It's trying to prevent you from being judged and rejected—which, at some point in your past, were real threats.

Question 3: "How old were you when you learned to do this?"

Often, Manager strategies formed in childhood or adolescence in response to specific situations.

You: "When did you start criticizing me like this?"

Inner critic: "When you were eight. When your dad yelled at you for not doing your homework perfectly. I learned that if I caught your mistakes first, maybe he wouldn't be so angry."

This helps you see that the Manager is using a child's logic. It's trying to solve an eight-year-old's problem with an eight-year-old's solution.

Question 4: "What do you need from me to be able to relax a little?"

This invites the Manager to collaborate with you rather than control you.

You: "What would you need from me to feel okay backing off the constant criticism?"

Inner critic: "I'd need to know you won't just become lazy or careless. I'd need to trust that you can handle feedback without falling apart."

Now you have information. This Manager needs reassurance that you (your adult Self) can handle criticism without being destroyed by it. It needs evidence that you're no longer eight years old and powerless.

Talking Back Without Fighting

Once you understand what a Manager is afraid of, you can respond from Self.

This isn't arguing. It's not trying to convince the Manager it's wrong. It's offering a new perspective and building trust.

You might say: "I get it. You learned to criticize me before anyone else could because that felt safer. That made sense when I was a kid. But I'm an adult now. I can handle feedback. I can make mistakes and learn from them without being destroyed. I don't need you to be this harsh to keep me safe. I've got this."

The Manager probably won't trust you immediately. That's okay. This is a relationship you're building. It takes time.

But each time you do this—each time you recognize a Manager, get curious about its fears, and respond from Self—you're strengthening two things:

1. The Manager's trust that you can lead
2. Your capacity to stay in Self even when parts are activated

Common Managers and Their Fears

Let's look at some common Manager parts and what they're typically protecting you from.

The Perfectionist

What it does: Drives you to be flawless in everything. No mistakes allowed.

What it's afraid of: Criticism, shame, rejection. "If you're not perfect, people will see you're inadequate and reject you."

What it needs from you: Evidence that you can handle imperfection. Reassurance that your worth isn't tied to perfect performance.

The People-Pleaser

What it does: Says yes when you mean no. Prioritizes others' needs over yours. Avoids conflict.

What it's afraid of: Abandonment, anger, rejection. "If people are unhappy with you, they'll leave. You'll be alone."

What it needs from you: Evidence that you can tolerate people being upset. Reassurance that you can set boundaries and survive the discomfort.

The Analyzer

What it does: Keeps you in your head, intellectualizing everything. Turns feelings into problems to solve.

What it's afraid of: Feelings. "If you feel too much, you'll be overwhelmed. If you're vulnerable, you'll get hurt."

What it needs from you: Evidence that feelings aren't dangerous. Reassurance that you can feel and not fall apart.

The Hypervigilant Scanner

What it does: Constantly watches for danger. Anticipates worst-case scenarios. Never relaxes.

What it's afraid of: Being caught off-guard. "If I stop scanning, something bad will happen and you won't see it coming."

What it needs from you: Evidence that you can handle surprises. Reassurance that you don't need constant surveillance to be safe.

The Over-Functioner

What it does: Stays busy, productive, helpful. Never stops. Never asks for help.

What it's afraid of: Being seen as weak, needy, or burdensome. "If you need help, people will see you're not capable. You have to handle everything alone."

What it needs from you: Evidence that asking for help isn't dangerous. Reassurance that needing support doesn't make you weak.

The Worksheet: A Compassionate Dialogue with Your Inner Critic

Let's make this concrete. Choose one Manager that's been particularly active lately—probably your inner critic, since it's the most common one.

Find a quiet time when you can access your anchor and get into Self. Then work through these questions. Write down your answers.

Part 1: Identify the Manager

1. What does this part say to you most often? (Write down the actual words it uses, even if they're harsh.)

2. When is this part most active? (What situations trigger it?)

3. How does your body feel when this part is active? (Tight chest? Racing heart? Tension? Shutdown?)

Part 2: Get Curious

From Self (calm, curious, compassionate), ask the part these questions and write down what comes:

4. "What are you trying to do for me?"

5. "What are you afraid would happen if you stopped doing this?"

6. "How old were you when you started doing this job?"

7. "What was happening in my life when you formed?"

Part 3: Respond from Self

8. What does this part need to hear from you? (Not arguing, not dismissing—what reassurance or perspective can you offer?)

9. What evidence can you give this part that you (as an adult with resources) can handle what it's afraid of?

10. What might you need to do to help this part start to trust you?

Part 4: Experiment

11. Choose one small situation this week where this Manager usually runs the show. Can you notice it activating, anchor yourself in Self, and make a different choice?

Example: If your inner critic activates after a work mistake, can you notice it, anchor yourself, and respond with self-compassion instead of self-attack?

Write down what happens when you try this.

Elena's Story: Befriending the Perfectionist

Elena, a 28-year-old graphic designer, was exhausted. Her perfectionism was crushing her. She'd redo projects five, six, seven times. She'd stay up until 2 AM tweaking details no one else would notice. She couldn't send an email without reading it ten times.

She hated this part of herself. She'd tried to "just stop being a perfectionist" countless times. It never worked. The harder she fought it, the louder it got.

When she learned to work with it as a part, everything shifted.

She got anchored in Self and asked her Perfectionist: "What are you trying to do for me?"

The answer surprised her: "I'm trying to make sure no one can criticize you. I'm trying to make your work so good that no one can reject it."

Elena dug deeper: "What are you afraid would happen if my work wasn't perfect?"

The Perfectionist's answer: "People would see that you're a fraud. They'd realize you're not as talented as they think. They'd reject you. You'd lose everything."

Then Elena asked the key question: "When did you start doing this?"

The answer came with a memory: Elena was twelve. She showed her mom a drawing she'd worked hard on. Her mom barely looked at it and said, "That's nice, honey. You could do better, though."

The Perfectionist formed in that moment. Its logic: "If you do better—if you do everything perfectly—maybe mom will actually see you. Maybe she'll be proud. Maybe you'll be enough."

Twenty-eight-year-old Elena could see that this was a twelve-year-old's solution to a twelve-year-old's pain.

From Self, Elena said to her Perfectionist: "I understand why you do this. You were trying to get mom's approval. That made sense. But I'm not twelve anymore. I don't need mom's approval to know I'm good at my work. I can handle feedback. I can make mistakes and my worth doesn't disappear. You don't have to work this hard anymore. I've got this."

The Perfectionist didn't believe her immediately. But Elena kept having this conversation. Every time the Perfectionist ramped up, Elena would anchor, get into Self, and remind it: "I've got this. You can rest."

Gradually, the Perfectionist started to relax. Elena's work was still excellent—but she wasn't destroying herself to achieve it.

What Happens When Managers Don't Trust You

Sometimes Managers won't step aside. Even when you're kind to them, even when you explain that you can handle things, they refuse to let go of control.

This usually means one of two things:

1. You're not actually in Self.

If you're trying to negotiate with a Manager from sympathetic activation or dorsal shutdown, the Manager perceives that you're not capable of leading. You're asking it to trust you while you're clearly not okay.

Solution: Go back to your anchor. Get more deeply into ventral. Try again when you're genuinely in Self.

2. The Manager is protecting an Exile that's too scared.

If there's a wounded part (an Exile) that's terrified and overwhelmed, the Manager won't step aside because it knows letting you near that Exile will be painful.

Solution: You need to work with the Manager even more. Reassure it that you won't force your way to the Exile. You'll go slowly. You'll make sure the Exile feels safe before you approach it. This builds trust.

The Daily Practice

Working with Managers isn't a one-time conversation. It's an ongoing relationship.

Here's the daily practice:

Morning: Set an intention.

"Today, when my Managers activate, I'm going to notice them from Self instead of being them."

Throughout the day: Notice and name.

Every time you catch a Manager driving—the inner critic, the perfectionist, the people-pleaser—pause. Name it.

"There's my Perfectionist again."

If you have time, anchor yourself and ask it: "What are you afraid of right now?" Just listen. You don't need to fix anything. Just acknowledge it.

Evening: Reflect.

"What Managers were most active today? What were they protecting me from? How did I respond—from Self or from another part?"

This practice builds the muscle of Self-leadership. Over time, your Managers learn to trust you. They start to relax. They don't have to control everything because they see that you're capable of leading.

What You're Actually Doing

This process might sound simple. Maybe even too simple.

But what you're doing is profound: **You're reparenting yourself.**

Your Managers formed when you were young and needed protection. They're still using strategies that made sense for that younger version of you.

Now, your adult Self is stepping in and saying, "I see you. I understand why you're doing this. But I'm the adult now. I can handle this. You can rest."

This is Internal Family Systems therapy in action. You're not trying to eliminate parts or suppress them. You're updating them. You're helping them recognize that the threat they're guarding against is no longer present.

And as your Managers begin to trust you, space opens up. Space to be spontaneous, to be vulnerable, to rest, to feel.

That space is where healing happens.

But there's one more type of protector we need to address—the reactive ones, the emergency responders. Your Firefighters.

The Core Understanding

Your Manager parts aren't enemies attacking you—they're protectors trying desperately to keep you safe using strategies that once worked. The inner critic that seems cruel is actually trying to protect you from criticism or rejection by others. The perfectionist isn't trying to torture you; it's trying to prevent shame or failure. These parts developed when you were younger and vulnerable, and they're still using childhood logic to solve adult problems.

The shift from being controlled by Managers to leading them happens through recognition and curiosity, not combat. When you can notice "There's a part of me that's criticizing" instead of "I'm such a failure," you've created space between Self and part. From that space, you can get curious about what the Manager fears and what it needs from you to relax its grip.

Building trust with your Managers is gradual work that requires consistent practice from your Compassionate Core. Each time you anchor yourself in Self and compassionately address a Manager's fears, you're demonstrating that your adult Self can actually handle what the Manager is trying to control. Over time, as these parts begin to trust your leadership, they relax their rigid strategies and allow space for spontaneity, vulnerability, and healing.

Chapter 7: Work with Your Rescuers (The Firefighters)

You're doing it again.

Scrolling through your phone at midnight, exhausted but unable to stop. Or reaching for food when you're not hungry. Or snapping at someone who didn't deserve it. Or disappearing into your head, checked out, gone.

And afterward, the shame hits. "Why did I do that? I know better. What's wrong with me?"

Here's what you need to understand: **Nothing is wrong with you.**

What you're experiencing is a Firefighter—an emergency response part trying to help you the only way it knows how.

Firefighters are the reactive protectors. While Managers try to prevent pain before it happens, Firefighters jump in *after* pain has surfaced. Their job is simple: make it stop. Right now. By any means necessary.

The strategies Firefighters use often create problems. But the parts themselves aren't problems. They're desperate attempts at self-protection.

This chapter teaches you how to work with Firefighters—not by suppressing them or fighting them, but by understanding what they're trying to rescue you from.

Understanding Firefighter Logic

Imagine your house is on fire.

A firefighter shows up and sprays water everywhere. They break windows. They cut holes in your roof. They make a mess. They cause damage.

But they're not trying to destroy your house. They're trying to save it. The damage is collateral—necessary to prevent total loss.

Your Firefighter parts work the same way.

When an Exile (a wounded part holding pain) gets triggered and surfaces, it feels unbearable. The pain is too big, too overwhelming, too intense. Your system perceives it as an emergency—a fire that needs to be extinguished immediately.

So a Firefighter jumps in with whatever works fastest: numbing, distracting, dissociating, rage, bingeing, risky behavior. The Firefighter's goal isn't to heal the pain. It's to stop you from feeling it right now.

The method causes problems later (the binge, the hangover, the damaged relationship, the shame). But in the moment, the Firefighter is just trying to save you from drowning in unbearable feelings.

Why Fighting Firefighters Doesn't Work

Most approaches to changing unwanted behaviors focus on stopping them.

"Just don't binge." "Stop procrastinating." "Control your anger." "Don't drink."

This doesn't work because you're trying to eliminate a protector without addressing what it's protecting you from.

When you try to suppress a Firefighter, one of three things happens:

1. The Firefighter gets stronger.

It sees your attempt to stop it as dangerous. If you won't let it use its strategy, how will you survive the pain? So it doubles down. The urge gets more intense. The behavior gets more compulsive.

2. A different Firefighter takes over.

You stop binge-eating, but suddenly you're dissociating constantly. You quit drinking, but now you're lashing out in rage. Different strategy, same job—just rescue you from pain.

3. You temporarily succeed through willpower, then collapse.

You white-knuckle it for a while. You use sheer force to suppress the behavior. But you can't sustain that forever. Eventually, the Exile's pain builds up, and the Firefighter breaks through with even more intensity.

None of these outcomes are actual healing.

The only way to work with Firefighters is to understand what they're protecting you from and address that.

Common Firefighters and What They're Rescuing You From

Let's look at typical Firefighter strategies and the pain they're trying to prevent you from feeling.

Numbing Behaviors (binge-eating, excessive screen time, scrolling, binge-watching)

What the Firefighter does: Creates distraction or alters your state so you don't have to feel what's underneath.

What it's rescuing you from: Loneliness, emptiness, worthlessness, grief, or other unbearable feelings.

Substance Use (alcohol, drugs, excessive caffeine or sugar)

What the Firefighter does: Chemically alters your state to provide relief.

What it's rescuing you from: Anxiety, shame, trauma memories, social discomfort, or emotional pain.

Dissociation (spacing out, feeling unreal, watching yourself from outside)

What the Firefighter does: Disconnects you from your body and the present moment.

What it's rescuing you from: Overwhelming fear, memories of trauma, or feelings too intense to bear in your body.

Rage or Lashing Out

What the Firefighter does: Channels pain into anger, which feels more powerful than vulnerable feelings.

What it's rescuing you from: Hurt, rejection, helplessness, or shame. Anger covers more vulnerable feelings.

Self-Harm or Risk-Taking

What the Firefighter does: Creates a different kind of pain or intensity to override emotional pain.

What it's rescuing you from: Emotional pain that feels more unbearable than physical pain. Or it's trying to feel *something* when you're too numb.

Compulsive Sexual Behavior

What the Firefighter does: Uses intensity, connection, or physical sensation to override emotional pain or numbness.

What it's rescuing you from: Loneliness, shame, emptiness, or trauma-related feelings.

Workaholism or Excessive Productivity

What the Firefighter does: Keeps you so busy that you don't have time or space to feel.

What it's rescuing you from: Feelings of worthlessness, fear of being alone with yourself, or avoidance of relationship issues.

The Pause and Pivot Practice

The most powerful skill you can develop with Firefighters is this: **catching them in the moment of activation, before you act on their impulse.**

This isn't about stopping them through willpower. It's about creating space between the impulse and the action—space where Self can show up and get curious.

Here's the practice:

Step 1: Notice the Urge

You feel the impulse rising. The urge to binge, to scroll, to dissociate, to lash out.

In that moment, name it: "There's a Firefighter activating."

Just naming it creates a tiny bit of space. You're observing the part instead of being the part.

Step 2: Pause

Don't act on the impulse yet. Just pause for 60 seconds.

This is the hardest part. The Firefighter wants immediate relief. Waiting feels intolerable.

But you're not suppressing it forever. You're just pausing long enough to get into Self.

Step 3: Anchor Yourself

Use one of your anchor practices from Chapter 5. Take a vagal sigh. Ground through your feet. Orient to your environment.

Get your nervous system into ventral, even just a little. Access Self—that calm, curious, compassionate presence.

This is essential. You can't work with a Firefighter when you're in sympathetic activation or dorsal shutdown. You need to be in Self.

Step 4: Get Curious

From Self, ask the Firefighter: **"What are you trying to rescue me from feeling right now?"**

Listen. The answer might come as words, as an image, as a felt sense in your body.

"I'm trying to rescue you from that loneliness you felt after your friend cancelled plans."

"I'm trying to rescue you from the shame that's surfacing about that mistake you made."

"I'm trying to rescue you from feeling how scared you are about that upcoming situation."

There's always something underneath. The Firefighter isn't random. It's reacting to pain.

Step 5: Acknowledge and Redirect

Once you understand what the Firefighter is protecting you from, you can respond.

First, acknowledge it: "Thank you for trying to help. I see you're trying to rescue me from this painful feeling. I get it."

Then, offer a different option: "But I'm going to try something else right now. I'm going to stay present with this feeling for a bit and see if I can handle it without numbing out. If it gets too intense, I'll come back to you."

This isn't rejecting the Firefighter. It's negotiating with it. You're saying, "I see why you're here, and I'm grateful. But let me try leading for a bit."

Step 6: Stay with the Feeling (Briefly)

Here's the radical part: You actually let yourself feel what the Firefighter was trying to prevent you from feeling.

Not forever. Not drowning in it. Just for a minute or two.

From Self, with your nervous system anchored, you can be present with uncomfortable feelings without being overwhelmed by them.

You might notice: "There's loneliness here. It's uncomfortable. But I can handle it. It's not going to destroy me."

Or: "There's shame here. It feels bad. But it's just a feeling. It will pass."

This is the healing moment. You're showing your Firefighter (and the Exile it's protecting) that you can be with difficult feelings without falling apart.

Over time, as you do this more, your Firefighters learn to trust you. They don't have to react so desperately because they see that you can handle what comes up.

The Firefighter's Message Exercise

Let's make this practical. Think of a Firefighter behavior you've engaged in recently—something you do when you're overwhelmed that you later regret.

Maybe it's scrolling your phone for hours. Maybe it's snapping at people. Maybe it's binge-eating or drinking or dissociating.

When you have time and space, work through these questions:

Part 1: Identify the Pattern

1. What's the Firefighter behavior? (Be specific. What exactly do you do?)

2. When does this happen most often? (What situations or triggers tend to activate this Firefighter?)

3. What do you usually feel right before the urge hits? (Or, if you feel nothing, what happened right before you went numb?)

Part 2: Understand the Rescue

4. If this Firefighter could talk, what would it say it's trying to do for you?

5. What feeling or experience is it trying to rescue you from? (Loneliness? Shame? Fear? Helplessness? Grief?)

6. When did you first start using this strategy? (How old were you? What was happening in your life?)

Part 3: What's Underneath

7. If you didn't numb/distract/rage/dissociate, what would you have to feel?

8. Is there an Exile (a younger, wounded part) that holds this feeling? (Can you sense a younger version of yourself that carries this pain?)

9. What is that Exile afraid would happen if it fully felt this feeling?

Part 4: Building a New Response

10. What does your Firefighter need to hear from you (from Self) to feel okay stepping back?

11. What evidence can you give it that you can handle uncomfortable feelings without falling apart?

12. Next time this Firefighter activates, what will you try instead? (What anchor practice? What way of staying present with the feeling?)

Michael's Story: Working with the Rage Firefighter

Michael, a 35-year-old teacher, had an anger problem. Or so he thought.

He'd snap at his partner over small things. He'd rage at other drivers. He'd lose his temper with his students. Afterward, he'd feel terrible—ashamed, guilty, like he was a bad person.

He'd tried anger management. He'd tried breathing exercises. Nothing stuck. The rage kept coming.

When he learned about Firefighters, everything made sense.

His rage wasn't the primary problem. It was a *reaction* to something underneath.

Michael started using the Pause and Pivot practice. The next time he felt rage rising—his partner left dishes in the sink again—he paused instead of exploding.

He anchored himself (grounding through his feet, vagal sigh). From Self, he asked his Rage Firefighter: "What are you rescuing me from?"

The answer surprised him: "I'm rescuing you from feeling helpless and disrespected."

Michael went deeper: "When did I start using rage this way?"

A memory surfaced: He was ten. His older brother used to bully him. Michael couldn't fight back—his brother was bigger, stronger. He felt helpless, humiliated.

But one day, Michael got so angry he fought back. His brother backed off. In that moment, Michael's system learned: Rage is power. Rage prevents helplessness.

Now, thirty-five-year-old Michael's Rage Firefighter jumped in anytime he felt disrespected or powerless. Dishes in the sink? That's disrespect. Rage kicks in.

From Self, Michael could see this was a ten-year-old's solution. Adult Michael didn't need rage to feel powerful. He could set boundaries, have conversations, handle discomfort without exploding.

He started talking to his Rage Firefighter: "I get why you do this. You learned that rage protects me from feeling helpless. That made sense when I was ten. But I'm not powerless anymore. I can handle disrespect without rage. I've got this."

The Rage Firefighter didn't believe him immediately. But Michael kept practicing. Pause. Anchor. Get curious. Stay with the underlying feeling (helplessness, disrespect) instead of covering it with rage.

Gradually, the rage episodes decreased. Not because Michael suppressed them, but because the Firefighter started to trust that Michael could handle things without needing rage as a shield.

When Firefighters Won't Back Down

Sometimes, even when you do everything right, a Firefighter won't step aside.

The urge is too strong. You can't pause. You act on the impulse.

This happens for a few reasons:

1. The Exile's pain is too intense.

If the underlying feeling is too overwhelming, the Firefighter will insist on its strategy. It's genuinely trying to save you from drowning.

Solution: You need to work with the Exile more directly. We'll cover this in the next chapter. For now, just know: If Firefighters are constantly active, there's deep pain underneath that needs attention.

2. You're not anchored enough in Self.

If you're trying to work with a Firefighter from sympathetic activation or dorsal shutdown, you don't have the capacity to stay with difficult feelings. The Firefighter knows this and won't let you near the pain.

Solution: Build your nervous system regulation capacity more. Practice your anchors daily. Strengthen your access to ventral before trying to work with intense Firefighters.

3. The Firefighter doesn't trust you yet.

Trust takes time. If you've spent years using Firefighter strategies, those parts won't trust that you can handle things differently after one conversation.

Solution: Keep showing up. Keep practicing the Pause and Pivot. Each time you successfully stay present with a difficult feeling without falling apart, you're building trust. It's cumulative.

Self-Compassion for When You "Fail"

You're going to act on Firefighter impulses sometimes. You're going to binge or dissociate or rage or numb out even after learning all this.

That's not failure. That's part of the process.

Your Firefighters have been doing their job for a long time. They're not going to retire overnight just because you learned a new framework.

When you act on a Firefighter impulse, here's what to do:

1. Don't shame yourself.

Shame just activates more Firefighters. Criticizing yourself for bingeing often leads to... more bingeing.

2. Get curious afterward.

"Okay, I just did the thing. What was I trying to rescue myself from? What feeling was too much?"

Even if you couldn't catch it in the moment, you can learn from it afterward.

3. Acknowledge the Firefighter's intention.

"Thank you for trying to help. I see you were trying to protect me from that painful feeling. Next time, I'm going to try staying present with it. But I appreciate that you're trying to help."

4. Recommit to the practice.

"Next time this comes up, I'm going to try the Pause and Pivot again. I'm learning. It's okay that I didn't get it this time."

This is how you build Self-leadership. Not through perfection. Through compassionate persistence.

Firefighters Are Not the Enemy

This is the most important thing to understand about Firefighters: **They're not the problem. They're a symptom of the problem.**

The problem is the Exiles—the wounded parts holding unbearable pain.

Firefighters are just trying to help. They're trying to keep you functional, keep you moving, keep you from being overwhelmed.

Their strategies cause problems. But their intention is protective.

So when you work with Firefighters, you're not trying to get rid of them. You're trying to:

1. Understand what they're protecting you from

2. Build their trust that you can handle difficult feelings

3. Offer alternative strategies that don't create collateral damage

As Firefighters begin to trust you, they relax. They don't have to react so desperately. They can let you (Self) lead.

And that creates space to do the deeper work—working with the Exiles those Firefighters have been protecting.

Which is exactly where we're going next.

The Essential Truth

Firefighters aren't enemies attacking you—they're emergency responders trying to save you from unbearable pain. When an Exile's feelings surface and threaten to overwhelm you, Firefighters jump in with whatever works fastest to stop the pain: numbing, bingeing, dissociating, raging. Their strategies cause problems, but their intention is always protective.

Fighting Firefighters through willpower or suppression doesn't work because you're trying to eliminate a protector without addressing what it's protecting you from. When you suppress one Firefighter strategy, another often takes its place, or the original one returns with even more intensity. The only effective approach is understanding what pain lies beneath the behavior and building the Firefighter's trust that you can handle those feelings.

The Pause and Pivot practice creates space between the Firefighter's impulse and your action—space where Self can get curious about what's underneath. By anchoring yourself in your Compassionate Core and asking "What are you trying to rescue me from feeling right now?" you can discover the Exile's pain the Firefighter is protecting. As you demonstrate repeatedly that you can stay present with difficult feelings without falling apart, your Firefighters gradually learn to trust your leadership and relax their desperate strategies.

Chapter 8: Safely Witness Your Wounded Parts (The Exiles)

You've been avoiding this.

Not consciously maybe. But your whole system has been designed around not going here—not feeling the pain your Exiles hold.

Your Managers have been controlling your life to prevent these wounds from being touched. Your Firefighters have been reacting desperately when the wounds surface anyway.

All of that protection, all of that effort, all of that avoidance—it's been about keeping you away from the Exiles.

The scared child. The humiliated teenager. The abandoned one. The ashamed one. The parts of you that hold the pain you couldn't process when it happened.

This is the chapter where we finally go there. But we're going carefully. We're going slowly. And we're only going when your system is ready.

Because here's the truth: **This is the healing part.**

Working with Managers and Firefighters creates safety and builds trust. But working with Exiles is where transformation actually happens. This is where the pain that's been driving your whole system finally gets witnessed, held, and released.

Why You've Been Avoiding Exiles

Your Exiles hold unbearable feelings.

Not just sadness or fear—*unbearable* sadness, *unbearable* fear. Feelings that, when they first happened, were too big for you to handle. So your system did what it had to do: It locked those feelings away in Exile parts and threw every protective strategy at keeping them there.

Think about it. If you're a child and something terrible happens—abuse, neglect, betrayal, loss—you can't fully process that. You don't have the resources. You don't have the support. You don't have the nervous system capacity.

So your system splits off those feelings and assigns them to a part. That part gets exiled—pushed into the basement of your psyche, locked behind layers of protection.

Your Managers make sure you never get close to that basement door. Your Firefighters react if you accidentally open it.

This system worked. It kept you functional. It kept you alive.

But it also kept you stuck. Because those Exiles are still there, still holding that pain, still frozen in the past.

And until they're witnessed and unburdened, they'll keep affecting your present.

What Exiles Need

Exiles don't need you to fix them or save them or explain away what happened to them.

They need something simpler and more profound: **They need to be seen.**

They need someone (your Self) to witness their pain without judgment, without trying to make it go away, without being overwhelmed by it.

They need to tell their story. They need to be believed. They need to know that what happened to them wasn't their fault.

And they need to be retrieved from the past—to be shown that the terrible thing isn't happening anymore, that they're not still trapped in that moment.

This is what "unburdening" means in Internal Family Systems (Schwartz, 1995). It's not forgetting the past. It's releasing the Exile from being frozen in it.

The Prerequisites for Exile Work

You cannot do this work until three conditions are met.

Condition 1: Your nervous system must be regulated.

You need to be in ventral vagal—in your Compassionate Core. If you try to access Exiles while you're in sympathetic activation or dorsal shutdown, you'll either re-traumatize yourself or disconnect from the feelings entirely.

This is why we spent Chapter 5 on anchoring. Without that foundation, Exile work isn't safe.

Condition 2: Your protectors must give permission.

Your Managers and Firefighters have been guarding these Exiles for years. They won't let you near them unless they trust that you can handle it.

This is why we spent Chapters 6 and 7 on working with protectors. You needed to build trust first.

If your protectors still feel strongly that you shouldn't access an Exile, respect that. They know something you don't. Come back to working with them. Build more trust. Try again later.

Condition 3: You must be in Self.

Not a Manager trying to "fix" the Exile. Not a Firefighter trying to numb the pain. Self—calm, curious, compassionate, courageous.

Only Self can hold an Exile's pain without being overwhelmed by it or trying to make it go away.

If you're not in Self, stop. Anchor yourself. Get back to Self. Then proceed.

The Process: Witnessing an Exile

When all three conditions are met—you're regulated, your protectors have given permission, and you're in Self—you can begin the witnessing process.

This is best done in a safe, quiet space where you won't be interrupted. Give yourself at least 30 minutes.

Step 1: Access the Exile

Ask your Managers and Firefighters: "Is it okay if I talk to the part that holds [specific feeling or memory]?"

If they say yes, invite that Exile forward. You might say: "Part that feels [scared/ashamed/abandoned], I'd like to get to know you. Would you be willing to show yourself to me?"

Notice what comes. It might be:

- An image of your younger self

- A felt sense of emotion in your body

- A memory

- Just a knowing that the part is there

Don't force it. If the Exile doesn't want to show itself, respect that. Your protectors are still unsure. Come back another time.

Step 2: Notice How You Feel Toward the Exile

This is critical. Check: Are you in Self?

Ask yourself: "How do I feel toward this part right now?"

If you feel **curious, compassionate, calm, or open**—you're in Self. Continue.

If you feel **critical, scared, numb, or you want to fix/save/rescue the part**—you're not in Self. Another part has jumped in between you and the Exile.

If that happens, talk to the part that jumped in: "I appreciate you trying to protect me, but I need you to step back so I can be with this Exile. Can you do that?"

Usually, if you're patient and respectful, protective parts will step aside.

Step 3: Ask the Exile to Show You What Happened

From Self, say to the Exile: "I'm here. I'm listening. Will you show me or tell me what happened?"

Let the Exile share its story. This might come as:

- Memories

- Images

- Feelings in your body

- Words or thoughts

You don't need to relive the trauma in detail. You just need to witness it. Stay present but don't merge with the Exile's feelings— you're with the part, not consumed by it.

If it gets too intense, pause. Use your anchors. Get back into Self. Then return.

Step 4: Validate and Reassure the Exile

Once the Exile has shared, respond from Self:

"I see you. I hear you. I believe you. What happened to you was real and it wasn't your fault."

This might sound simple. But for an Exile that's been hidden and blamed for years, this is profound.

You might say:

- "You were just a child. You didn't deserve that."

- "You were so scared and alone. No one should have to feel that way."

- "It makes sense that you felt [ashamed/terrified/worthless]. Anyone in that situation would feel that way."

Let the Exile receive this. It might take time.

Step 5: Ask What the Exile Needs

"What do you need from me?"

The Exile might need:

- To be held or comforted

- To be told it's safe now

- To be retrieved from the past (shown that the trauma is over)

- To be protected or defended

- To be given permission to express anger or sadness

Do whatever the Exile needs, imaginally. If it needs to be held, imagine holding your younger self. If it needs to be protected, imagine standing between your younger self and whoever hurt them.

This is symbolic work, but it's deeply powerful. You're giving the Exile what it needed then but didn't get.

Step 6: Retrieve the Exile from the Past

This is the "unburdening" step (Schwartz, 1995).

Ask the Exile: "Do you know that this isn't happening anymore? That you're not still in that situation?"

Often, Exiles are frozen in time. They don't know that the trauma ended. They're still experiencing it as if it's happening now.

If the Exile is stuck in the past, you need to show it the present.

You might say: "That happened a long time ago. It's [current year] now. You're not [age of trauma] anymore. You're safe. The danger is over."

Invite the Exile to come with you to the present. Imagine taking your younger self by the hand and walking out of the traumatic situation into your current life.

Show the Exile: "Look, we're okay now. We survived. We're here."

Step 7: Ask if the Exile is Ready to Release the Burden

Exiles carry burdens—beliefs formed during trauma. Beliefs like:

- "I'm worthless"

- "I'm unlovable"

- "I'm not safe"

- "It's my fault"

- "I can't trust anyone"

These beliefs made sense in the context of the trauma. But they're not true in the present.

Ask the Exile: "Are you ready to let go of the belief that [burden]?"

If yes, ask: "How do you want to release it?"

The Exile might want to:

- Imagine the burden leaving through light or water

- Hand it to you to throw away

- Burn it, bury it, dissolve it

Use whatever imagery feels right to the Exile. This is symbolic, but it works. You're updating the Exile's core belief.

Step 8: Invite the Exile to a New Role

Once unburdened, the Exile doesn't need to stay in exile.

Ask: "Now that you've released that burden, what would you like to do? What role would you like to have in my life?"

Often, Exiles become sources of joy, creativity, playfulness, or connection once they're no longer carrying trauma.

A scared child Exile might become a part that feels safe playing, exploring, being curious.

An abandoned teenager Exile might become a part that can form genuine connections with others.

The Exile doesn't disappear. It integrates. It becomes a healthy part of your system, no longer frozen in pain.

The Worksheet: The Unburdening Process

This is advanced work. Don't rush it. Only do this when you feel ready, when your protectors have given permission, and when you can stay anchored in Self.

Work through these questions slowly. Take breaks. Use your anchors as needed.

Part 1: Preparation

1. Which Exile do you want to work with? (What feeling or memory does it hold?)

2. Have you asked your protectors for permission? (Do they feel okay with you accessing this Exile right now?)

3. Are you in Self? (Check: Do you feel calm, curious, compassionate toward the Exile? Or do you feel critical, scared, or numb?)

Part 2: Witnessing

4. When you invite the Exile forward, what do you notice? (An image? A feeling? A memory? A sense of a younger you?)

5. What is the Exile trying to show you or tell you?

6. What happened to this part? (You don't need graphic details. Just the essence of what this part experienced.)

Part 3: Validation

7. From Self, what do you want to say to this Exile? (Validation, reassurance, apology for not seeing it sooner?)

8. What does the Exile need to hear from you?

Part 4: Unburdening

9. What burden (belief) is this Exile carrying? ("I'm worthless," "I'm unsafe," "It's my fault," etc.)

10. Is the Exile ready to release this burden?

11. How does it want to release it? (Imagery: light, water, fire, handing it away, etc.)

12. Once the burden is released, what shifts? (How does the Exile feel now?)

Part 5: Integration

13. Now that it's unburdened, what role does this part want in your life?

14. What does it need from you going forward?

15. How do you feel toward this part now?

Anna's Story: Unburdening the Shame Exile

Anna, a 41-year-old lawyer, carried deep shame. She couldn't pinpoint where it came from exactly—it just felt like a constant background hum. "I'm defective. Something's wrong with me."

This shame drove everything. Her perfectionism (Manager trying to prove she wasn't defective). Her people-pleasing (Manager trying to prevent rejection). Her tendency to shut down during intimacy (Firefighter protecting her from vulnerability).

When Anna felt ready—after months of anchoring practice and working with her protectors—she decided to meet the Exile that held her shame.

She got regulated. She asked her protectors for permission. They hesitated, but eventually agreed.

From Self, Anna invited the Exile forward: "Part that feels all this shame, I want to meet you. Will you show yourself?"

An image came: Anna at age seven, standing in her bedroom, feeling... wrong. Bad. Like there was something fundamentally broken about her.

Anna (from Self) asked: "What happened?"

The Exile showed her: Anna's parents fighting. Her mother, drunk and angry, screaming at her father. Anna trying to intervene, trying to make it better. Her mother turning on her: "This is your fault. You ruin everything. I wish you were never born."

Seven-year-old Anna internalized that message completely. "I'm the problem. I ruin everything. I'm defective."

Adult Anna, from Self, could see the truth: That was her mother's pain, her mother's addiction talking. It had nothing to do with seven-year-old Anna.

From Self, Anna said to the Exile: "That wasn't true. You were a child. You didn't ruin anything. Mom was sick. She was in pain. What she said wasn't about you. You deserved love, not blame."

The Exile wept. Anna stayed present with it, holding the feelings without being overwhelmed.

Then Anna asked: "Do you know that you're not seven anymore? That you're not in that room?"

102

The Exile didn't. It was still frozen in that moment.

Anna said: "Come with me. Let me show you."

She imagined taking seven-year-old Anna by the hand and walking her out of that bedroom, into adult Anna's life now. "Look, we're okay. We survived. We're strong. We're good at our job. We have people who care about us. We made it."

The Exile could see it. The relief was palpable.

Anna asked: "Are you ready to let go of the belief that you're defective?"

Yes.

"How do you want to release it?"

The Exile imagined the shame as a heavy, dark rock. She handed it to adult Anna, who threw it into the ocean. Gone.

Without the shame, the Exile felt light. Free. She could play, be curious, feel joy.

Anna asked: "What role do you want now?"

The Exile said: "I want to remind you that you're allowed to be imperfect. You're allowed to be human."

This wasn't a one-time fix. Anna still had moments of shame. But they were less intense, less frequent. And when shame came up, Anna could recognize it: "That's the old burden trying to come back. But I don't have to carry it anymore."

The Exile was no longer running her life.

Going Slowly

Some people can do this work relatively quickly. Others need years.

There's no timeline. There's no "should."

If you have multiple Exiles (and most people with complex trauma do), you work with them one at a time. You don't need to unburden every Exile to start healing. Even working with one can shift your entire system.

And some Exiles aren't ready. Some need more time, more trust, more reassurance from protectors.

That's okay. Healing isn't linear. It's not a checklist. It's a relationship—between you (Self) and all your parts.

When This Work is Too Much

If attempting Exile work activates intense Firefighters—if you immediately dissociate, binge, rage—that's a sign you're not ready yet.

Go back to working with Managers and Firefighters. Build more trust. Strengthen your nervous system regulation. Practice anchoring daily.

There's no shame in not being ready. This is the deepest, hardest work. It requires resources and capacity that take time to build.

Consider working with a therapist trained in IFS or trauma work. A skilled guide can help you navigate this safely.

What Happens After Unburdening

When an Exile is unburdened, the system shifts.

The Managers that were protecting that Exile can relax. They don't have to control so desperately.

The Firefighters that were reacting when that Exile surfaced can rest. They don't have to rescue you from pain that's no longer there.

You have more access to Self. More capacity to be present, to feel, to connect.

You're not "cured." You're not suddenly trauma-free. But you're no longer carrying the same weight. You're no longer living from a place of pain that happened years ago but still feels like it's happening now.

You're here. In the present. With all your parts working together, led by your Compassionate Core.

And that changes everything.

The Heart of the Work

Your Exiles hold the unbearable feelings from your past—pain that was too overwhelming to process when it happened, so your system locked it away and built layers of protection around it. These aren't just uncomfortable feelings; they're the core wounds that drive your entire protective system. Your Managers and Firefighters have spent years keeping you away from these Exiles because they genuinely believed the pain would destroy you.

Exile work is where actual healing happens, but it requires three non-negotiable conditions: a regulated nervous system, permission from your protectors, and your presence as Self. Without these, attempting to access Exiles leads to retraumatization or dissociation. This is why all the previous work—anchoring, befriending Managers, understanding Firefighters—was necessary preparation.

The unburdening process isn't about forgetting trauma or minimizing what happened. It's about witnessing the Exile's pain from your Compassionate Core, validating what happened, and helping the Exile understand that it's no longer trapped in that moment. When Exiles release their burdens and recognize they're safe now, they integrate into your system as sources of vitality rather than frozen repositories of pain. Your entire protective system can finally relax, and Self can lead your life from the present rather than constantly reacting to a past that won't let go.

Chapter 9: Living from Your Compassionate Core

You've learned the framework. You've practiced the skills. You understand your nervous system states, your parts, your patterns.

Now comes the real challenge: **living this.**

Because it's one thing to do these practices in a quiet moment when you have time and space. It's another thing entirely to use them when life is happening—when you're triggered at work, when your partner says something that activates your Exiles, when you're overwhelmed and exhausted and your Firefighters are screaming for relief.

This is where theory becomes practice. This is where you learn to lead your life from Self—consistently, repeatedly, imperfectly.

This chapter shows you how.

What Self-Led Living Actually Means

Living from your Compassionate Core doesn't mean you're always calm.

It doesn't mean you never get triggered. It doesn't mean your parts disappear or stop having opinions. It doesn't mean you're suddenly immune to stress or pain.

What it means is this: **When life activates your nervous system or your parts, you notice it, and you lead your response.**

Instead of being hijacked by a sympathetic activation spiral, you catch it. You anchor. You respond from Self.

Instead of your inner critic running the show, you notice it's active and lead from compassion instead.

Instead of a Firefighter making decisions for you, you pause, get curious, and make a choice from Self.

You're not perfect. You're not always successful. But you're leading more often than you're being led. And that makes all the difference.

The Integration Sequence

When something triggers you, here's what happens in real-time:

1. Something happens (the trigger)

Your partner forgets to do something they promised. Your boss criticizes your work. You get an unexpected bill. Someone cancels plans.

2. Your nervous system reacts

Before you even consciously register what happened, your autonomic system shifts. You might activate (sympathetic) or shut down (dorsal).

3. Parts get activated

Your Managers jump in to control the situation. Your Firefighters stand ready to numb or distract if needed. Your Exiles might surface with feelings from the past.

At this point, most people react from parts and states, not from Self.

But you're learning something different. Here's the sequence that lets you lead from Self:

Step 1: Notice Your State

The moment you feel activated—heart racing, thoughts spiraling, anger rising, numbness descending—name it.

"My nervous system is in sympathetic right now."

or

"I'm in dorsal shutdown right now."

This creates space. You're observing your state instead of being your state.

Step 2: Notice Your Parts

Once you've identified your nervous system state, check: Which parts are active?

"My inner critic is loud right now."

"My people-pleasing Manager wants me to apologize even though I didn't do anything wrong."

"My Rage Firefighter wants to lash out."

Again, you're observing. You're not these parts. You have these parts, and they're activated.

Step 3: Use Your Anchor

Before you do anything else, anchor yourself.

Use whatever practice works best for you in that state. Vagal sigh. Grounding through your feet. Orienting to your environment.

The goal is to shift back toward ventral, even just a little. To access some Self.

This might take 30 seconds. It might take 5 minutes. Don't skip this step. You can't lead from Self if you're not in Self.

Step 4: Get Curious

Once you're anchored (even partially), get curious about what's happening.

Ask yourself:

- "What am I actually feeling underneath this reaction?"
- "What am I afraid of right now?"

- "What part is most active, and what does it need?"

If it's a Manager: "What are you trying to protect me from?"

If it's a Firefighter: "What are you trying to rescue me from feeling?"

If it's an Exile: "What old feeling is this touching?"

Curiosity shifts you further into Self. Judgment keeps you in parts.

Step 5: Lead with Compassion

From Self, decide how you want to respond.

Not how your parts want you to respond. Not what your nervous system's automatic reaction is. What *you* (Self) choose to do.

Maybe you choose to set a boundary. Maybe you choose to have a difficult conversation. Maybe you choose to feel your feelings without acting on them. Maybe you choose to ask for help.

Whatever you choose, you're choosing from Self—from that calm, clear, compassionate presence—not from reactivity or protection.

This is Self-led living.

A Real-Time Example

Let's walk through how this looks in a real situation.

Situation: Your friend cancels plans at the last minute. Again.

Immediate reaction:

Your nervous system activates (sympathetic). Your chest tightens. Anger rises. Thoughts spiral: "They don't care about me. I'm not important to them. Why do I even bother?"

Step 1: Notice your state.

"I'm activated right now. Sympathetic. My heart is racing and I'm getting angry."

Step 2: Notice your parts.

"There's my Catastrophizer Manager—it's telling me this means they don't care. And there's an Exile underneath that feels unimportant and rejected."

Step 3: Anchor.

You take two vagal sighs. You ground through your feet. You look around your room, orienting to your actual environment.

Your nervous system shifts slightly. You're not completely calm, but you're more present.

Step 4: Get curious.

"What's really happening here? My friend cancelled. That's disappointing. The Catastrophizer is trying to protect me from being blindsided by rejection. The Exile is feeling that old 'I don't matter' wound."

Step 5: Lead with compassion.

From Self, you decide: "I'm not going to respond to the text right now. I need some time. But later, I'm going to tell my friend that this pattern bothers me. I'm going to set a boundary from a place of self-respect, not from reactivity."

You also talk to your Exile: "I see you. You feel unimportant. That makes sense based on what happened in the past. But this situation isn't the same. My friend cancelling doesn't mean I don't matter."

You've led from Self. You didn't suppress your feelings. You didn't react from them. You were with them and chose your response.

Making Self-Led Decisions

Self-led decisions feel different from part-led decisions.

Part-led decisions feel:

- Pressured, urgent, compulsive
- Like you "have to" or "should"

- Driven by fear, shame, or avoidance
- Like you'll regret them later

Self-led decisions feel:

- Spacious, clear, grounded
- Like a choice you're making freely
- Aligned with your values
- Like you can stand behind them

When you're making a decision—big or small—check in with yourself:

"Am I deciding this from Self, or from a part?"

If you're not sure, ask:

- "What am I afraid would happen if I didn't do this?"
- "Is this decision driven by a Manager trying to control something?"
- "Is this decision driven by a Firefighter trying to avoid something?"

If yes, pause. Anchor. Get into Self. Then decide.

Building This into Daily Life

Integration isn't something you do once. It's something you practice constantly.

Here's how to make this a daily habit:

Morning: Set your intention.

"Today, I'm going to practice noticing when I'm not in Self and anchoring back."

Throughout the day: Micro-practices.

Every time you feel activated, even slightly, run the sequence: Notice state. Notice parts. Anchor. Get curious. Lead with compassion.

At first, you'll only catch it after you've already reacted. That's fine. You're building awareness.

Over time, you'll catch it in the moment. Eventually, you'll catch it before you react.

Evening: Reflect.

"When did I lead from Self today? When did I react from parts? What do I want to do differently tomorrow?"

This isn't about judgment. It's about building the skill.

When You Can't Access Self

Some days, you won't be able to access Self no matter what you do.

You're too activated. Too shut down. Too overwhelmed. Your protectors are too loud. Your Exiles are too raw.

When that happens, **don't force it.**

Instead, do basic self-care:

- Rest if you can
- Use your anchors even if you can't access full ventral
- Be gentle with yourself
- Ask for help if you need it

And recognize: This is information. If you can't access Self, something needs attention. Maybe you're overwhelmed and need to lighten your load. Maybe an Exile needs witnessing. Maybe your system is exhausted and needs real rest.

Living from Self doesn't mean being in Self constantly. It means coming back to Self more quickly when you get knocked out of it.

Carlos's Story: Integration in Action

Carlos, a 44-year-old project manager, used to be ruled by his Manager parts.

He'd overwork himself constantly (Manager trying to prove his worth). He'd avoid difficult conversations (Manager trying to prevent conflict). He'd analyze every decision to death (Manager trying to control outcomes).

And when his Managers failed—when he got overwhelmed—his Firefighters would take over. He'd shut down emotionally, zone out in front of the TV for hours, disconnect from everyone.

After learning this framework, Carlos started practicing the integration sequence.

First situation: His director questioned his timeline for a project.

Old pattern: Catastrophize ("I'm going to get fired"). Work until midnight revising the timeline. Snap at his wife when he got home.

New pattern: Notice the activation (sympathetic). Notice the Catastrophizer Manager ("You're not good enough. You have to fix this right now"). Anchor (vagal sigh, grounding). Get curious ("What's this Manager afraid of? Failure. Shame. Being seen as incompetent."). Lead from Self ("This feedback isn't catastrophic. I can have a conversation with my director about realistic timelines. I don't have to prove my worth by overworking.")

He still felt anxious. The Manager didn't disappear. But he led the response from Self instead of letting the Manager run the show.

Second situation: A few weeks later, Carlos felt overwhelmed. He'd been working intensely, and he just wanted to check out.

Old pattern: Binge-watch TV until 2 AM, ignore his wife's attempts to connect, feel worse the next day.

New pattern: Notice the urge (Firefighter wanting to numb). Pause. Anchor. Get curious ("What am I trying to avoid feeling? Exhaustion. Loneliness. Fear that I can't keep up."). Lead from Self ("I'm exhausted. I need rest. But numbing out isn't real rest. I'm going to tell my wife I need some downtime, and I'm going to actually rest—maybe read, maybe take a bath, maybe go to bed early.")

Was it perfect? No. He still watched more TV than he planned. But he didn't completely check out. He stayed somewhat present. He made a choice from Self rather than being hijacked by a Firefighter.

Over months of practice, Carlos spent more and more time in Self. His Managers relaxed because they saw he could lead. His Firefighters were less active because his Exiles weren't being triggered as often.

He wasn't cured. He still had hard days. But he was leading his life, not being led by his parts.

The Lifelong Practice

Here's what nobody tells you: This work doesn't end.

You don't "graduate" from having parts. You don't reach a point where you're always in Self and never get triggered.

Living from your Compassionate Core is a lifelong practice, just like physical health is a lifelong practice.

You'll have setbacks. You'll have periods where you're back in old patterns. You'll have days where Self feels completely inaccessible.

That's not failure. That's being human.

The difference is, you now have tools. You understand what's happening. You know how to come back to Self when you've been knocked out of it.

And each time you practice—each time you notice, anchor, get curious, and lead—you're strengthening neural pathways. You're building capacity. You're teaching your system that Self can lead.

That's the work. It's simple. It's not easy. But it's worth it.

What's Possible

When you live more consistently from Self, certain things become possible that weren't before:

You can have relationships without constantly bracing for betrayal.

When your Managers aren't controlling every interaction and your Exiles aren't getting triggered constantly, you can actually be present with people. You can be vulnerable without feeling like you're going to die. You can trust, cautiously, because your Self can handle disappointment if it comes.

You can make choices based on your values, not your fears.

When your protectors aren't running the show, you can choose based on what actually matters to you—not what keeps you safe, not what avoids pain, but what aligns with who you want to be.

You can feel your feelings without being destroyed by them.

When your Self can hold your Exiles' pain, you don't have to avoid every difficult emotion. You can be sad without spiraling into depression. You can be angry without raging. You can be scared without panicking.

You can rest without guilt.

When your Managers trust that you can handle your life, they don't have to drive you constantly. You can rest, actually rest, because you're not trying to prove your worth every moment.

You can fail without falling apart.

When your worth isn't tied to perfect performance (because your Exiles have been unburdened of that belief), you can make mistakes, learn from them, and move on. Failure doesn't confirm your deepest fear that you're defective. It's just information.

You can be yourself.

This is the big one. When you're not constantly performing for your Managers, numbing out with your Firefighters, or being haunted by your Exiles, you can just... be.

You can show up as you are. Imperfect, messy, human, enough.

That's what living from your Compassionate Core makes possible.

The Practice Never Ends, and That's Okay

You're going to have to do this sequence—notice, anchor, get curious, lead—for the rest of your life.

That might sound exhausting. But consider the alternative: Being led by your protectors and your pain for the rest of your life.

This way is better. Harder sometimes, but better.

Because this way, you're living your life. Not the life your trauma dictates. Not the life your protectors think you need to survive. Your life, led by your Self, guided by your values, connected to what actually matters.

You've spent so long being led by parts that were just trying to keep you alive.

Now you get to lead—from your Compassionate Core, from Self, from that place in you that was never broken and never needed fixing.

Welcome home.

Bringing It All Together

Living from your Compassionate Core means leading your responses instead of being led by automatic reactions. When triggers happen—and they will—you move through a consistent sequence: notice your nervous system state, identify which parts are active, use your anchor to access Self, get curious about what's underneath the reaction, and then choose your response from that grounded place. This isn't about achieving perfect calm; it's about returning to Self more quickly after you're knocked out of it.

Self-led decisions feel spacious and aligned with your values, while part-led decisions feel urgent, pressured, and driven by fear or avoidance. Building the capacity to distinguish between these requires daily practice—setting morning intentions, catching yourself throughout the day when you're not in Self, and reflecting each evening on where you led and where you were led. This isn't something you master once; it's a lifelong practice of strengthening the neural pathways that allow Self to guide your life.

What becomes possible as you strengthen this practice is profound: relationships without constant bracing, choices based on values rather than fears, the ability to feel without drowning, rest without guilt, failure without collapse, and the freedom to simply be yourself. You'll still get triggered, your parts will still activate, and some days Self will feel completely unreachable. But you now have a map back to your Compassionate Core, and each time you use it, you're building the internal leadership that lets you live from presence rather than protection, from choice rather than compulsion, from who you actually are rather than who trauma taught you to be.

Chapter 10: Handling Triggers and Setbacks in Real-Time

You're going to get stuck.

Not if. When.

There will be moments when nothing you've learned seems to work. When you can't access Self no matter how hard you try. When your protectors refuse to budge. When you're so activated or shut down that you can't even remember what ventral vagal means, let alone find it.

This isn't failure. This is part of the process.

Healing isn't a straight line. You don't steadily improve until you reach some finish line where you're permanently fixed. You have good days and terrible days. Breakthroughs and breakdowns. Moments of clarity and moments where you forget everything you've learned.

What makes the difference isn't avoiding these stuck moments. It's knowing how to navigate them when they happen.

This chapter is your troubleshooting guide. Real-time solutions for the most common situations where you'll find yourself spinning, stuck, or completely lost.

Think of this as the manual you pull out when everything else has stopped working.

When You Feel Numb (Dorsal Shutdown)

You're sitting there, staring at nothing. Someone asks how you're doing and you genuinely don't know. You can't feel anything. Not sad, not anxious, not even really there.

This is dorsal vagal shutdown. Your system has pulled the plug to protect you from overwhelm.

The problem: When you're in shutdown, you can't access your parts, you can't feel your feelings, and most of the practices you've learned require some degree of presence that you simply don't have right now.

So what do you actually do?

Step 1: Accept Where You Are

First, stop fighting it.

The worst thing you can do when you're numb is judge yourself for being numb. That just activates more shame, which pushes you further into shutdown.

Say this instead: "I'm in dorsal shutdown right now. My system is protecting me from something. That's okay. This will pass."

Acceptance doesn't mean you like it. It means you stop adding suffering on top of suffering.

Step 2: Gentle Mobilization

You need to climb back up the nervous system ladder—from dorsal to sympathetic to ventral. That means you need to gently add some activation without overwhelming yourself.

Try these, one at a time:

Move your body. Not intense exercise—that can be too much. Just movement. Stand up and shake out your arms and legs for 30 seconds. Take a short walk, even if it's just around your house. Do some gentle stretches.

The goal is to get some blood flowing, some sensation back in your body. Movement says to your nervous system: "We're here. We're alive. We're okay to engage."

Create sensation. Hold an ice cube in your hand. Splash cold water on your face. Take a hot shower. Eat something with a strong taste— sour, spicy, intensely flavored.

Physical sensation can pull you back into your body when you've disconnected from it.

Connect with something outside yourself. Call a friend. Pet your dog. Watch something that makes you feel something—a movie that usually moves you, music that typically stirs emotion.

Sometimes you can't generate feeling from inside yourself. You need to borrow it from outside until your system comes back online.

Make sound. Hum. Sing. Talk out loud to yourself. The vibration of sound through your vocal cords stimulates your vagus nerve and can help shift your state (Porges, 2017).

Step 3: Don't Force Feelings

When you're numb, there's an impulse to force yourself to feel. "I should be feeling something about this. What's wrong with me?"

Don't do that. You're numb because feelings felt too big. Forcing them before your system is ready will just push you back into shutdown.

Instead, work on presence. Just being in your body, noticing sensations, engaging with your environment. Feelings will return when your nervous system feels safe enough to allow them.

Step 4: Check for Hidden Overwhelm

Sometimes numbness is a sign that you've been pushing too hard, doing too much, feeling too much. Your system has hit its limit and shut down to protect you.

Ask yourself: "Have I been overwhelmed lately? Have I been processing a lot? Have I been ignoring my need for rest?"

If yes, the solution isn't to push through the numbness. It's to actually rest. Let your system recover. Do easy, comforting things. Lower your expectations for a few days.

What Doesn't Work When You're Numb

Don't: Try to do complex parts work. You can't access your parts when you're shut down.

Don't: Meditate or sit in stillness. That often makes shutdown worse because you're just sitting with nothing.

Don't: Isolate completely. Connection can help pull you out, even if you don't feel like connecting.

Don't: Use substances to try to feel something. That just adds more confusion to your system.

Laura's Example: Finding the Way Out of Shutdown

Laura, a 39-year-old therapist (yes, therapists deal with this too), found herself completely numb after a particularly intense week at work. She'd been holding space for other people's pain all week, and her system had had enough.

Saturday morning, she woke up feeling... nothing. Not tired, not rested, not sad, not relieved that the week was over. Nothing.

Old Laura would have panicked or judged herself. New Laura recognized it: "I'm in shutdown. My system needs a break."

She didn't try to process anything. She didn't try to feel her feelings. Instead, she went for a walk—not a purposeful "healing walk," just walking. She let her dog pull her around the neighborhood. She felt the sun, noticed the trees, moved her body.

After 20 minutes, she felt a tiny bit more present. Not much, but something.

She came home and made herself a strong cup of coffee—the taste and caffeine created sensation. She called her sister and just chatted about nothing important—connection without pressure.

By afternoon, she wasn't fully back online, but she was no longer completely numb. She could feel some things. Not everything, but enough.

She let herself rest for the remainder of the weekend without trying to "fix" the numbness. By Monday, her system had recovered and she felt relatively normal again.

When You're in a Panic (High Sympathetic Activation)

Your heart is pounding. You can't breathe right. Your thoughts are racing—catastrophizing, spinning, jumping from one worst-case scenario to another. Your body is screaming at you that something terrible is about to happen.

But nothing is actually happening. You're safe. Your nervous system just doesn't know that.

This is high sympathetic activation. Full-blown panic.

Step 1: Name It

In the middle of panic, your brain is convinced the threat is real. You need to remind it that this is your nervous system, not reality.

Say out loud (or in your head if you're in public): "This is a panic attack. This is my sympathetic nervous system. This is not real danger. This will pass."

Naming it creates a tiny bit of distance between you and the panic. You're observing it, not fully merged with it.

Step 2: Vagal Sigh—Immediately

This is your first-line tool for panic. The double-inhale, long exhale pattern we covered in Chapter 5.

Do it 3-5 times in a row. Don't worry about whether it's "working." Just do it.

This pattern physiologically activates your ventral vagal brake on your sympathetic system (Balban et al., 2023). It's not magic, but it works more often than not.

Step 3: Orient to Your Environment

Your brain is convinced there's danger. Show it there isn't.

Look around. Name 5 things you can see. Say them out loud if you can.

"I see a chair. I see a window. I see a plant. I see a book. I see a cup."

This pulls you out of your internal panic and into your actual environment. It shows your nervous system: "Look, we're in a room. Nothing is attacking us. We're okay."

Step 4: Ground Through Your Body

Feel your feet on the floor. Press them down. Feel the support underneath you.

Put your hand on something solid—a wall, a table, the ground. Feel its texture, its temperature, its solidity.

This reminds your system that you have a body, you're in a place, you're not floating in a void of terror.

Step 5: Ride the Wave

Panic attacks peak and then subside. They don't last forever, even though it feels like they will.

Research shows that panic attacks typically peak within 10 minutes and then start to decrease (Craske & Barlow, 2007). Your job is to ride that wave without adding more fear on top of the fear.

Don't fight the panic. Don't try to make it stop immediately. Just breathe through it. "This is temporary. I can handle 10 minutes of discomfort. I've done it before. I'll do it again."

Step 6: Identify the Trigger (Later)

Don't try to analyze why you're panicking while you're panicking. Just get through it.

But later, when you've calmed down, get curious: "What triggered that? What was my system responding to?"

Often, panic attacks aren't random. Something activated an Exile's fear—a situation that reminded your system of past danger. Understanding the trigger helps you work with it proactively next time.

What Doesn't Work When You're Panicking

Don't: Try to think your way out. Your prefrontal cortex is offline. Logic doesn't work right now.

Don't: Tell yourself to "calm down." That just adds frustration on top of panic.

Don't: Avoid whatever situation triggered the panic going forward. Avoidance makes panic worse over time.

Don't: Believe the catastrophic thoughts. They're not predictions—they're symptoms of activation.

James's Example: Panic in a Meeting

James, a 31-year-old marketing manager, felt panic rising in the middle of a presentation to executives. His boss had questioned one of his data points, and suddenly James's heart was racing, his vision was narrowing, and he couldn't think straight.

Old James would have pushed through, which usually made it worse, or excused himself and felt ashamed later.

New James recognized it: "Sympathetic activation. Not real danger. Just my nervous system."

He took a vagal sigh—disguised as just a deep breath—while pretending to think about the question.

He glanced around the room, orienting. These were colleagues, not threats. He was standing on solid ground.

He said, "Good question. Let me pull up the source for that," which gave him 30 seconds to ground himself while he navigated to the data.

By the time he found the information, the peak of the panic had passed. He answered the question, finished the presentation, and later recognized what had triggered him: His boss questioning him activated an Exile that carried shame about being wrong, which activated massive fear of being exposed as incompetent.

He worked with that Exile later. But in the moment, he just got through the panic without making it worse.

When a Protector Won't Step Aside

You're trying to work with an Exile. You're regulated, you're in Self, you've asked your protectors for permission. But one of them refuses.

Maybe your inner critic keeps jumping in, criticizing you for trying this work. Maybe your intellectual Manager keeps pulling you into analysis. Maybe a Firefighter keeps dissociating you every time you get close to the pain.

The protector isn't being difficult. It's doing its job. It genuinely believes letting you near that Exile will hurt you.

So what do you do?

126

Step 1: Don't Force It

The biggest mistake people make is trying to push past a resistant protector.

"I know you're scared, but I need to do this, so please move."

That doesn't work. The protector digs in harder. Its whole job is to protect you, and you're asking it to stop doing its job.

Instead, slow down. Respect the protector's boundary. "Okay, you don't want me going there right now. I hear you."

Step 2: Get Curious About the Fear

Ask the protector: "What are you afraid would happen if you stepped aside?"

Listen carefully. The answer might be:

"You'll fall apart and not be able to function."

"The pain will be too much and you'll get stuck in it."

"You'll be vulnerable and someone will hurt you."

"You'll realize how bad it was and you won't be able to handle that."

The protector has a specific fear. You need to understand it before you can address it.

Step 3: Build Trust Slowly

Once you understand the fear, respond from Self—not trying to convince the protector it's wrong, but offering reassurance.

"I get why you're scared. That pain was really big when I was younger. But I'm an adult now. I have resources. I have tools. I can handle this. And I won't go too fast. I'll go slowly, and if it gets too intense, I'll stop."

This isn't a one-time conversation. Building trust takes multiple interactions. You might need to have this conversation with the protector several times before it relaxes.

Step 4: Work with the Protector Instead

If the protector still won't budge, don't force it. Work with the protector itself.

"Okay, you don't feel ready for me to access that Exile yet. Can you tell me more about yourself? When did you start doing this job? What was happening in my life?"

Often, understanding the protector's history helps. These parts formed for a reason. Honoring their story builds relationship.

Step 5: Check If You're Actually in Self

Sometimes protectors won't step aside because you're not actually in Self. Another part is pretending to be Self.

Check: How do you feel toward this protector?

If you feel frustrated, annoyed, impatient—you're not in Self. Another part (probably a Manager that wants to "fix" things quickly) has jumped in.

If that's the case, talk to that part first. "I appreciate you wanting to help, but you need to step back so Self can lead."

Only from genuine Self—calm, curious, compassionate—can you build trust with resistant protectors.

Step 6: Consider the Timing

Maybe the protector is right. Maybe now isn't the time.

Maybe you've been under a lot of stress. Maybe your life circumstances don't support deep processing right now. Maybe you need to build more nervous system capacity first.

Trust the protector's wisdom. Come back to the Exile later, when conditions are better.

What Doesn't Work with Resistant Protectors

Don't: Try to overpower them with willpower. That makes them more rigid.

Don't: Ignore them and force your way to the Exile. That's retraumatizing.

Don't: Judge them as "resistance" or "the problem." They're protectors doing their job.

Don't: Give up entirely. Just because they're not ready now doesn't mean they won't be ready later.

Nina's Example: The Protector That Wouldn't Budge

Nina, a 36-year-old artist, wanted to work with an Exile that held grief about her mother's death. But every time she tried to access that grief, her Analyzer Manager would jump in and intellectualize everything.

She'd get close to tears, and suddenly she'd be thinking about the stages of grief, analyzing her emotional response, explaining to herself why she felt this way.

She tried asking the Analyzer to step aside. It wouldn't.

Finally, she got curious: "Analyzer, what are you afraid would happen if I actually felt this grief?"

The answer: "You'll drown in it. You won't be able to stop crying. You'll fall apart and you won't be able to paint, and if you can't paint, you'll lose yourself."

Nina (from Self) could see the fear was real. This part believed grief would destroy her.

She didn't try to convince it otherwise. Instead, she said: "I understand. You think I can't handle the grief. What would you need to see to believe I can handle it?"

The Analyzer said: "I'd need to see you feel some grief and still be okay afterward. Still be functional."

So Nina made a deal: "Okay, let me feel the grief for just 2 minutes. You can time it. After 2 minutes, if I'm not okay, you can jump back in. But give me 2 minutes."

The Analyzer agreed.

Nina let herself cry for 2 minutes. It was intense. But after 2 minutes, she was still there. Still breathing. Still herself.

The Analyzer saw it. "Okay, you handled that. Maybe you can handle more."

Over time, the Analyzer relaxed more and more. It learned that grief didn't destroy Nina. And eventually, it stepped aside enough for Nina to fully unburden that Exile.

When You Can't Remember What to Do

Sometimes you get so triggered, so activated or shut down, that you completely forget everything you've learned.

You know you have tools. You know there's a process. But in the moment, your brain is offline and you can't access any of it.

This is completely normal. Your prefrontal cortex goes offline when your nervous system is in extreme states (Arnsten, 2009). Executive function—the part of your brain that plans, remembers, chooses—stops working properly.

The solution: Prepare for this in advance.

Create a crisis card. Write down your top 3-5 anchoring practices on a card or in your phone. When you're dysregulated and can't think, you can pull out the card and follow the instructions without having to remember.

Example:

1. Take 3 vagal sighs

2. Ground through feet—feel the floor

3. Name 5 things I can see

4. Hand on heart—"I'm here, I'm okay"

5. Call [trusted person's name]

Keep it simple. Keep it concrete. Keep it accessible.

Tell someone you trust. If you have a partner or close friend, tell them: "When I'm really dysregulated, I might not be able to access my tools. If you notice that, can you gently remind me? Just say, 'Maybe try your anchors?' or 'Want to do a vagal sigh together?'"

External support can bridge the gap when your internal resources are temporarily unavailable.

When You Have a Complete Meltdown

You will have meltdowns. Days where everything falls apart. Where you act from your most reactive Firefighters, say things you regret, do things that feel like huge steps backward.

This is not the end of your progress. This is part of the process.

After a meltdown:

1. Don't spiral into shame. You had a hard moment. You're human. Shame just activates more protectors and makes everything worse.

2. Return to basics. Don't try to do advanced parts work. Just get regulated. Use your anchors. Get your nervous system back to baseline.

3. Repair if needed. If you hurt someone during your meltdown, apologize and repair the relationship. Take responsibility without drowning in shame.

4. Get curious (later). Once you're calm, investigate: "What triggered that? What Exile got activated? What was my system trying to protect me from?"

5. Recommit. "Okay, I had a meltdown. That happens. I'm going to keep practicing. One meltdown doesn't erase all the progress I've made."

The Reality of Nonlinear Healing

You're going to have setbacks. You're going to have days where you feel like you've learned nothing. You're going to have moments where your old patterns come roaring back.

This doesn't mean you're not healing. This means you're healing in the messy, nonlinear way that healing actually happens (Herman, 1997).

Progress in trauma recovery looks more like a spiral than a straight line. You circle back to old issues at deeper levels. You have breakthroughs, then consolidation periods that feel like plateaus. You take two steps forward, one step back, three steps forward, two steps back.

The trajectory is upward. But the path isn't straight.

What matters isn't avoiding setbacks. What matters is how you respond to them. Do you use them as evidence that you're hopeless? Or do you use them as information, as opportunities to practice self-compassion, as proof that you're human?

Your choice.

Quick Reference Guide

When numb: Move body, create sensation, don't force feelings, check for overwhelm

When panicking: Name it, vagal sigh, orient to environment, ground through body, ride the wave

When a protector won't budge: Don't force, get curious about fears, build trust slowly, check if you're in Self, consider timing

When you forget everything: Use crisis card, reach out for support, return to basics

After a meltdown: Avoid shame, regulate first, repair if needed, get curious later, recommit

Keep this guide somewhere accessible. You will need it.

The Truth About Getting Stuck

Getting stuck isn't a sign you're doing it wrong. Getting stuck is part of doing it right. It means you're in the arena, trying, practicing, engaging with your healing instead of avoiding it. You can't get stuck doing something you're not attempting.

Every time you get stuck and find your way out, you're building resilience. You're proving to your nervous system and your parts that you can handle difficulty. You're creating evidence that Self can lead, even when things get hard.

The goal isn't to never get stuck. The goal is to trust that when you do get stuck, you have tools to work with it. You're not helpless anymore. You're not the person you were when the trauma happened. You have resources, you have awareness, you have Self.

That changes everything.

Chapter 11: From Survivor to Self

There's a moment that happens in healing that nobody talks about.

It's not dramatic. It's not a breakthrough or a revelation. It's quieter than that.

You're doing something ordinary—making coffee, driving to work, talking to a friend—and you notice: You feel... okay. Not ecstatic. Not "healed." Just okay.

And then you realize: This is new. This ease. This absence of constant background fear. This feeling like you're actually in your life instead of watching it from behind glass.

You're not managing symptoms. You're not white-knuckling your way through the day. You're just... living.

That's the moment you realize: You're not just surviving anymore. You're becoming yourself.

The Shift from Survivor to Self

For years, maybe decades, your identity has been shaped by survival.

Survivor of trauma. Survivor of abuse. Survivor of neglect. You've worn survival like armor, and it's kept you safe. It's helped you make sense of your struggles. It's given you a framework for understanding why you are the way you are.

But there comes a point where survival isn't enough. Where you don't just want to survive—you want to live.

This shift from survivor to Self isn't about denying what happened. It's not about pretending the trauma didn't matter or doesn't still affect you sometimes.

It's about refusing to let survival be your only story.

Survivors are defined by what happened to them. Self is defined by who you choose to be.

This distinction matters. When you're in survivor mode, your past runs your present. Your trauma makes your decisions. Your protectors lead your life. Your Exiles' pain colors everything.

When you're living from Self, you acknowledge the past without being controlled by it. You have protectors, but they don't run the show. You have wounds, but they don't define you.

You're here. Now. Choosing.

What Living from Self Actually Looks Like

Living from Self isn't some perfect state where you're always calm and wise and compassionate.

It's messier than that. More human than that.

Living from Self means:

You still get triggered, but you notice it faster and return to yourself sooner.

You still have anxious days, but they don't spiral into weeks of panic.

You still have parts that activate, but you can observe them instead of being them.

You still make mistakes, but you don't collapse into shame about them.

You can feel your feelings—all of them—without being destroyed by them or numbing them out.

You can connect with people without constantly bracing for betrayal.

You can rest without guilt, play without shame, succeed without waiting for the other shoe to drop.

You make choices based on your values instead of your fears.

You trust yourself, mostly. Not perfectly, but enough.

You're here. Present. Embodied. Alive in a way you weren't before.

The Three Dimensions of Living from Self

As you move from survivor to Self, three dimensions of your life begin to open up: connection, creativity, and purpose. These aren't separate goals you achieve—they're natural expressions of a nervous system that feels safe and a Self that's been freed to lead.

Connection

Trauma teaches you that connection is dangerous.

People hurt you. People leave. People betray. So you learned to disconnect, to protect yourself, to stay safe behind walls.

But humans are wired for connection (Porges, 2011). We literally need it to regulate our nervous systems. Isolation is itself a form of suffering.

Living from Self means you can start to risk connection again— carefully, gradually, with discernment.

What this looks like:

You can be vulnerable with safe people without feeling like you're going to die.

You can ask for help without feeling like a burden.

You can receive care without immediately pushing it away or feeling like you owe something.

You can set boundaries without apologizing for having needs.

You can disagree with someone without the relationship ending.

You can let people see you—actually see you, not the performed version—and trust that you'll survive if they don't like everything they see.

This doesn't mean connecting with everyone or trusting blindly. Living from Self includes the wisdom to know who's safe and who isn't. You're not naive. You're discerning.

But you're not assuming everyone will hurt you either. You're willing to find out.

Creativity

Trauma shuts down creativity.

When you're in survival mode, your brain is focused on threat detection and protection. There's no bandwidth for exploration, play, curiosity, or making things just because you want to.

Exiles hold pain, but they also hold qualities that got shut down along with the pain—spontaneity, joy, imagination, wonder (Schwartz, 1995).

As your Exiles get unburdened, as your protectors relax, those qualities come back online.

What this looks like:

You have ideas again. Not just anxious thoughts or problem-solving, but actual ideas—things you want to try, make, explore.

You can engage in activities just for enjoyment, not because they're productive or serve a purpose.

You notice beauty. Colors look brighter. Music moves you. Small moments feel meaningful.

You want to create things—art, writing, music, gardens, businesses, relationships, experiences. Not because you're trying to prove something, but because the impulse to create is part of being alive.

You take risks creatively. You try things you might fail at. You share your work even though it's imperfect.

Creativity isn't just about art. It's about engaging with life as something to explore rather than something to endure. It's about curiosity, experimentation, play.

When you're living from Self, creativity returns because your system finally has the safety and space to engage with the world as something other than a threat.

Purpose

When you're just surviving, your purpose is simple: Don't die. Don't fall apart. Get through the day.

That's a perfectly valid purpose when that's all you can manage.

But as you heal, something else emerges: You want your life to mean something. You want to contribute. You want to matter in ways that go beyond just managing symptoms.

Purpose doesn't have to be grand. It doesn't have to be changing the world or finding your "calling" (though it might be).

Purpose can be:

Showing up for the people you love in ways you couldn't before

Doing work that feels aligned with who you are

Contributing to something larger than yourself

Using what you've learned to help others who are struggling

Creating something meaningful—a family, a community, a body of work

Living in ways that reflect your values, not your fears

Living from Self means you have energy and attention for purpose because you're not spending all of it on survival.

You're not perfect. You still have hard days. But you have enough stability, enough inner safety, enough access to your Compassionate Core that you can think about what you want your life to be about.

The Paradox of Not Needing to Be Healed

Here's something strange that happens as you heal: You care less about being healed.

When you're in the thick of trauma, healing feels like the answer to everything. "If I could just heal, then I'd be happy. Then I'd have good relationships. Then I'd be successful. Then I'd finally be okay."

But as you actually heal, you realize: Being okay doesn't require being perfectly healed. Being okay is something you can access right now, in this moment, even with your history, even with your remaining struggles.

You stop waiting to be fixed before you start living.

You stop putting your life on hold until you're "better."

You engage with what's here—the messy, imperfect, still-healing version of yourself—and you find that this version is enough to build a life with.

This is the paradox: **You heal more when you stop making healing your entire identity and purpose.**

When you're obsessed with healing, you're still organized around your trauma. When you're living from Self, you're organized around your values, your interests, your relationships, your purpose. Healing continues, but it's happening in the background while you're busy living.

What About the Hard Days?

Living from Self doesn't mean you never have hard days.

You'll still have times when your nervous system gets dysregulated. When old patterns come back. When you feel stuck again.

The difference is, you don't spiral into "I'm not healing" or "I'll never get better."

You recognize: "I'm having a hard day. My system is stressed. I need to use my tools and take care of myself."

Hard days become data, not evidence of failure. They tell you something needs attention—maybe you're overwhelmed, maybe an Exile needs witnessing, maybe you need rest.

But they don't erase your progress. They don't mean you're back at square one. They're just part of being a human who's been through trauma and is learning to live differently.

Letting Go of the Trauma Identity

This is one of the hardest parts of moving from survivor to Self: letting go of trauma as your primary identity.

Trauma has probably explained so much for you. It's given you a framework for understanding your struggles. It's connected you to communities of people who've been through similar things. It's even given you a certain kind of purpose—healing from trauma, helping others heal from trauma.

But at some point, organizing your entire life around trauma keeps you stuck in it.

You can acknowledge trauma without making it your whole story.

You can say: "Yes, that happened. Yes, it shaped me. Yes, it still affects me sometimes. And also, I am more than that. I am more than what happened to me. I am what I'm choosing now."

This doesn't mean abandoning the survivor community or pretending the trauma doesn't matter. It means expanding your identity beyond it.

You're a survivor, yes. And you're also an artist, a parent, a friend, a partner, a professional, a person with interests and hobbies and dreams. You're funny, or kind, or curious, or determined. You're a human being with a full, complex life that includes trauma but isn't only trauma.

Reclaiming that fullness is part of the healing.

Grace's Story: Building a Life

Grace, a 43-year-old social worker, spent her thirties focused on healing. Therapy, workshops, books, practices. She did the work. She processed her childhood trauma. She unburdened her Exiles. She learned to regulate her nervous system.

And it helped. She felt better. More stable. More present.

But at some point, she realized: "I'm spending all my energy on healing and no energy on living. I'm not creating anything. I'm not connecting much. I'm just... working on myself."

So she made a decision: She was going to build a life, even if she wasn't perfectly healed.

She started dating, even though her attachment patterns weren't totally resolved. She joined a pottery class, even though her perfectionist Manager had opinions about her imperfect bowls. She volunteered at an animal shelter, even though it stirred up Exile feelings about her own childhood neglect.

She still had hard moments. She still got triggered. She still needed to use her tools.

But she was living. Creating. Connecting. Engaging with the world as more than just a person healing from trauma.

And ironically, the more she focused on living, the more healing happened naturally. Her nervous system regulated more easily because she had positive experiences to regulate toward. Her parts relaxed because she was proving, day by day, that she could handle life.

She moved from survivor to Self not by trying harder to heal, but by daring to live before she felt completely ready.

A Letter of Compassion to All Your Parts

You've spent this entire book learning about your parts— understanding them, working with them, negotiating with them.

Now it's time to speak to them directly. From Self. With compassion for everything they've tried to do for you.

Dear Parts,

I see you. All of you.

Inner Critic, Perfectionist, People-Pleaser, Analyzer—my Managers. You've been working so hard, for so long, trying to keep me safe. You learned that if I was just good enough, perfect enough, careful enough, then maybe I wouldn't get hurt. You've been trying to control an uncontrollable world, and I know how exhausting that's been.

I see you. Thank you for trying to protect me. I don't need you to work this hard anymore. But I appreciate that you have.

Rage, Dissociation, Binge-Eater, Numb-Out—my Firefighters. You've jumped in to rescue me from pain I couldn't handle. When feelings got too big, when Exiles surfaced, when I thought I would break—you did whatever you had to do to get me through. Your strategies caused problems, but your intention was always to save me.

I see you. Thank you for not letting me drown. I'm learning to handle pain differently now. But I appreciate that you kept me alive when I didn't know how.

Scared Child, Ashamed One, Abandoned One, Hurt One—my Exiles. You've carried pain that was too big, too overwhelming, too much. You've held shame that wasn't yours. You've felt fear that no child should ever feel. You've been locked away, not because you were bad, but because the pain you carried felt like it would destroy me.

I see you. I'm so sorry you had to carry that alone for so long. I'm here now. I'm listening. I'm witnessing. You don't have to hold that burden anymore.

To all my parts: You formed in response to things that actually happened. You developed strategies that made sense at the time. You did the best you could with the resources available.

You are not the problem. You never were. You're survivors, just like me.

But I'm leading now. I'm here. I'm the adult. I'm the one with resources, with safety, with the capacity to handle what you've been protecting me from.

You don't have to do this alone anymore. You can rest. You can trust me.

I've got us. I've got this.

We're going to be okay. Not perfect. Not without struggle. But okay.

Thank you for keeping me alive until I could learn to live.

With deep compassion and gratitude,
Self

Writing Your Own Letter

At some point—maybe now, maybe later—write your own letter to your parts.

Use your own words. Address the specific parts you know. Thank them for what they've tried to do. Apologize for the times you've fought them or hated them. Offer them compassion and reassurance from Self.

This isn't just symbolic. This is relationship-building with the internal system that's been running your life. This is leadership— Self stepping up and saying, "I've got this."

You can write different letters to different parts. You can rewrite the letter as your relationship with your parts changes. You can read the letter out loud to yourself when you need to reconnect with Self.

This practice matters. It's a commitment to leading from your Compassionate Core, even when it's hard.

What Happens Next

You've reached the end of this book, but not the end of your healing.

The work continues. The practice continues. The relationship with your parts continues.

Some days will be easy. Some will be brutal. Some will be ordinary in ways that feel miraculous because ordinary used to be out of reach.

You'll forget what you've learned and have to relearn it. You'll get stuck and have to find your way out again. You'll have breakthroughs and setbacks and long stretches where nothing much changes.

That's the reality of healing. Not linear, not perfect, not finished.

But different. So different from where you started.

You're not the same person you were when you picked up this book. You have a map now. You have tools. You have awareness. You have Self.

You know how to find your Compassionate Core when you lose it. You know how to work with your parts instead of being run by them. You know how to befriend your nervous system instead of being at war with it.

That knowledge doesn't go away. It's yours now.

The Invitation

Here's what I want you to know as you close this book:

You are not broken.

You never were. You're a human being who survived difficult things using the resources available at the time. Those survival strategies made sense. They worked. They kept you alive.

And now you're learning to live, not just survive. You're learning to lead from Self instead of being led by protection and pain.

This is the bravest work you'll ever do. Not because it's dramatic or heroic, but because it requires showing up, day after day, practicing, failing, trying again, being patient with yourself, choosing compassion over criticism, trusting that you can handle what comes.

You're doing it. You're here. You're trying.

That's enough. You're enough.

Welcome home to yourself.

The journey from there to here has been long. The journey forward will have its own challenges. But you're not walking it alone anymore. You have Self. You have your Compassionate Core. You have the capacity to lead your life.

That changes everything.

Go live. Create. Connect. Choose. Build a life that reflects who you actually are, not who trauma taught you to be.

You deserve that life. You always have.

And now, finally, you have the tools to claim it.

What You Take Forward

You started this book stuck—knowing something was wrong, trying everything, but not understanding why nothing worked. Now you know. You can't heal your mind's parts until you regulate your body's state. You can't access your Compassionate Core when your nervous system is screaming danger. Integration requires both body and mind working together.

The path forward isn't about perfection. It's about practice. Daily anchoring. Noticing when parts are driving. Getting curious instead of judgmental. Building trust with your protectors. Gently witnessing your Exiles. Leading from Self more often than you're led by survival patterns. Some days you'll do this well. Some days you'll forget everything. Both are part of the process.

Living from Self means reclaiming your full humanity—not just the survivor, but the creator, the connector, the person with purpose. You'll still have trauma history. You'll still have parts. You'll still have hard days. But you're no longer defined by what happened to you. You're defined by who you choose to be right now, in this moment, with all your messy, imperfect, beautiful humanity. That's the real healing—not erasing the past, but refusing to let it run your present. You've learned how. Now go do it.

Reference

- Arnsten, A. F. T. (2009). Stress signalling pathways that impair prefrontal cortex structure and function. *Nature Reviews Neuroscience*, 10(6), 410–422.

- Balban, M. Y., Neri, E., Kogon, M. M., Weed, L., Nouriani, B., Jo, B., Holl, G., Zeitzer, J. M., Spiegel, D., & Huberman, A. D. (2023). Brief structured respiration practices enhance mood and reduce physiological arousal. *Cell Reports Medicine*, 4(1), 100895.

- Cozolino, L. (2017). *The neuroscience of psychotherapy: Healing the social brain* (3rd ed.). W. W. Norton & Company.

- Craske, M. G., & Barlow, D. H. (2007). *Mastery of Your Anxiety and Panic: Therapist Guide* (4th ed.). Oxford University Press.

- Dana, D. (2018). *The polyvagal theory in therapy: Engaging the rhythm of regulation*. W. W. Norton & Company.

- Dana, D. (2020). *Polyvagal exercises for safety and connection: 50 client-centered practices*. W. W. Norton & Company.

- Herman, J. L. (1997). *Trauma and recovery: The aftermath of violence—from domestic abuse to political terror*. Basic Books.

- Khurana, R. K., Watabiki, S., Hebel, J. R., Toro, R., & Nelson, E. (1980). Cold face test in the assessment of trigeminal-brainstem-vagal function in humans. *Annals of Neurology*, 7(2), 144–149.

- Levine, P. A. (1997). *Waking the tiger: Healing trauma.* North Atlantic Books.

- Neff, K. D., & Germer, C. K. (2018). *The mindful self-compassion workbook: A proven way to accept yourself, build inner strength, and thrive.* Guilford Press.

- Porges, S. W. (2004). Neuroception: A subconscious system for detecting threats and safety. *Zero to Three*, 24(5), 19–24.

- Porges, S. W. (2011). *The polyvagal theory: Neurophysiological foundations of emotions, attachment, communication, and self-regulation.* W. W. Norton & Company.

- Porges, S. W. (2017). *The pocket guide to the polyvagal theory: The transformative power of feeling safe.* W. W. Norton & Company.

- Schwartz, R. C. (1995). *Internal family systems therapy.* Guilford Press.

- Schwartz, R. C. (2021). *No bad parts: Healing trauma and restoring wholeness with the internal family systems model.* Sounds True.

- Schwartz, R. C., & Sweezy, M. (2019). *Internal family systems therapy* (2nd ed.). Guilford Press.

- van der Kolk, B. A. (2014). *The body keeps the score: Brain, mind, and body in the healing of trauma.* Viking.

www.ingramcontent.com/pod-product-compliance
Lightning Source LLC
Chambersburg PA
CBHW070800290326
41931CB00011BA/2089